W9-DID-963

AQUACISES®

Terri Lee's Water Workout™ Book

AQUACISES®

Terri Lee's Water Workout™ Book

TERRI LEE

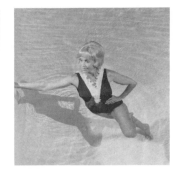

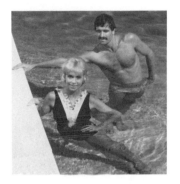

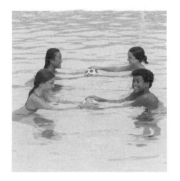

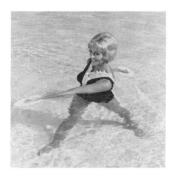

Library of Congress Cataloging in Publication Data

Lee, Terri.
　Aquacises : Terri Lee's water workout book.

　Includes index.
　1. Aquatic exercises.　I. Title.
GV505.L43 1984　　　613.7'1　　　83-13651
ISBN 0-8359-0152-1

First Printing 1984 - Reston Publishing Co.
Second Printing 1990 - Terri Lee

Copyright © 1984 by Terri Lee.

All rights reserved. No part of this book may be reproduced in any way, or
by any means, without written permission from the author.

Printed in the United States of America.

To my late parents who fostered and encouraged my lifelong love of the water and its fascinating inhabitants.

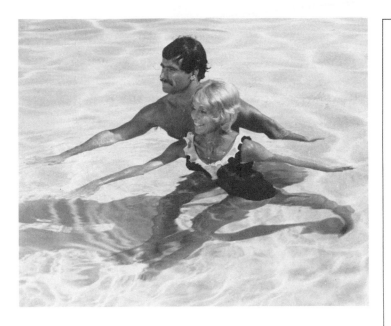

CONTENTS

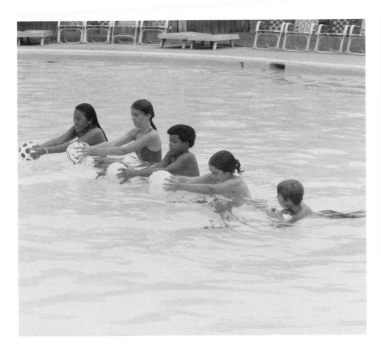

If your professional life has been involved with teaching others to swim, you may have been searching for a fresh and comprehensive text on aquatic exercise. Terri Lee, teacher and innovator, through her unique synthesis of the medical, physiological, and applied aspects of this increasingly popular area of aquatics, has taken time to write such a book.

Aquacises is literally a pharmacopoeia of body movements to be performed in the water. Components of physical or motor fitness such as flexibility, muscle strength, or coordination are identified with each exercise described. The exercises are applicable to those children and adults with medically defined disabilities. Aquacises can also be used by fitness-oriented swimmers who need a break in their lap-oriented routines. It is a text for everyone.

Anatomical and physiological benefits of swimming are well established. Terri Lee has extended the science of aquatic movement by adding an affective dimension. This is presented through the concept of perceived exertion. The reader is given the cornerstones for fitness development—namely frequency, intensity, and duration of exercise. Heart rate responses to exercise are to be used to monitor the intensity of the movements. Adding the concept of perceived exertion to an exercise routine emphasizes Terri Lee's concern for the safety of the exerciser.

Neither last nor overlooked is the fun element of exercise in the water. If there is to be a commitment to exercise throughout life, exercise must be enjoyable. A variety of movements with or without equipment or shared with other people is presented in

Aquacises. The combination of routines is limitless. Figures which accompany the text add immeasurably to the artistic quality of the book.

Only a lifetime of teaching and experimentation could have produced this text. Terri Lee's enthusiasm for aquatics is visible throughout. Her penchant for detail is commendable, and I recommend this text to you as the bridge between the science and art of aquatic exercise.

Karl G. Stoedefalke, Ph.D.
Exercise Scientist
The Pennsylvania University
and
Fellow, American College
of Sports Medicine

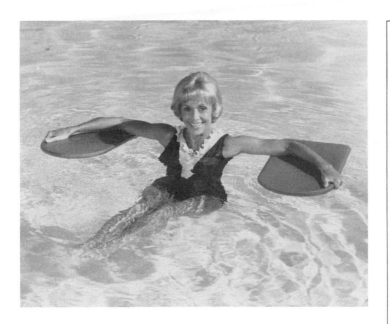

AQUACISES is a new, more analytical look at my original concepts for achieving fitness in the fascinating and inviting world of water.* All of the movements have been specially designed for the aquatic environment and are intended to provide:

1. A complete system of continuous, rhythmic activities, done with the head above the surface in a small area of any pool having waist-to-chest-deep water. (Many Aquacises can even be done in a lake or ocean.)
2. An exercise regimen that effectively increases muscular and cardiovascular fitness, yet is substantially free of adverse side effects such as muscle strains and ballistic impact to joints.
3. A multifaceted program that readily adapts to the fitness requirements of nearly everyone, including those individuals who need modified exercise regimens because of age, handicaps, or other limiting factors.
4. An interesting, sometimes challenging, and always enjoyable alternative to traditional aquatic activities—a welcome new dimension to swimming pool use.

Aquacises not only increase the strength, flexibility, and endurance of the body, but satisfy the child's love of play that exists in all of us. These exercises include hundreds of new movements, along with the most popular and effective ones

* My first book of aquatic exercise was published in 1969.

from the first book. During the intervening 13 years, all of the new movements and variations were tested on hundreds of enthusiastic students. Even heart rates were tested by the Human Performance Laboratory at Pennsylvania State University to confirm which categories of Aquacises contribute most to cardiovascular fitness.

Since most movements can be done at various energy levels according to individual needs, Aquacises are ideally suited to many applications such as:

1. Physical fitness and recreation programs for individuals exercising alone, or for high school, college, adult and family groups—even children's camps.
2. Postsurgical rehabilitation.
3. Pre- and postnatal conditioning
4. A change of pace from swimming laps.
5. A fun and enjoyable water-introduction course for non-swimmers (in a well-supervised environment).
6. Supplemental conditioning in conjunction with basic swimming, aquatic art, and synchronized swimming courses.
7. An adjunct to Water Workouts™ musical cassette programs to further increase one's fitness level.

Finally, it seemed only fitting to name these Aquacises after the dazzling array of creatures (both animal and plant) that inhabit the water or find sustenance there. After all, how could movements like the Trunkfish for the trunk, or Booby for you know what, be as much fun by any other name? I originally intended to correlate the Aquacise motion with the creature's mode of locomotion, mannerisms, or the name its image evokes, but this was frequently impossible. Therefore, some names were chosen simply because the animal or its name was especially appealing or unusual. In the Appendix, I have briefly summarized the most interesting characteristics of some of the less familiar children of the world's seas, lakes, rivers, and ponds. However, while the Appendix is based on authoritative data, it was prepared ''sole''-ly in the spirit of fun and is not to be construed as a scientific treatise.

What follows is my gift to you—the means to a life that is happier, healthier and, I sincerely hope, longer as well.

Terri Lee

ACKNOWLEDGMENTS

My heartfelt thanks to the many people who helped make this book possible. Among them:

My students—always an inspiration and some of my severest critics.

Mary Moffroid, R.P.T, Ph.D.; Karl Stoedefalke, Ph.D.; Howell Wright, physical educator; and William R. Moses, M.D., who generously contributed valuable expertise on various aspects of *Aquacises*.

J.B.S. who provided capable editorial help over the years and who skillfully inked my myriad pencil illustrations.

The many friendly and knowledgable curators at the Smithsonian Institution who answered my wide-ranging questions about aquatic creatures; and especially Dr. George Watson, curator of birds, who critiqued my copy on aquatic birds.

John Flanagan, a record holding Master swimmer and exemplary water-exercise enthusiast who kindly posed for photographs.

Dr. and Mrs. Vacit Y. Ozberkmen who so graciously made their beautiful pool available for numerous photography sessions.

The talented staff at Reston Publishing Company, particularly Laura Cleveland, my production editor, who also designed the interior of *Aquacises*.

ACKNOWLEDGMENTS

AQUACISES®
Terri Lee's Water Workout™ Book

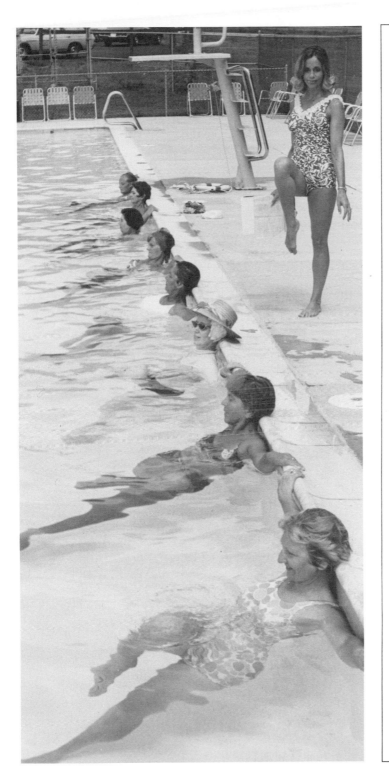

Part 1

GETTING TO KNOW AQUACISES®

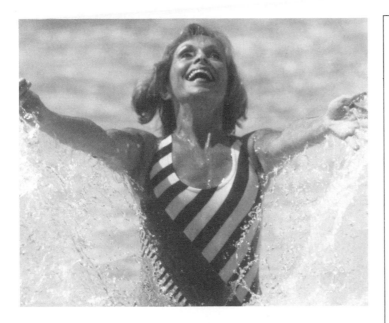

Chapter 1
WATER—OUR NATURAL HABITAT

"I am the sea, the sea is me."

So said Jacques Yves Cousteau, the celebrated French marine explorer, proclaiming both his love of the sea and his kinship with it—the same kinship many believe we all share.

We are all water beings living on a water planet. Just as the oceans cover over 70% of the earth's surface, fluids make up over 70% of the weight of our body (even more in newborn babies). This "sea of life" may be our heritage from remote aquatic ancestors—one that links us to the sea which, some think, is our original mother. Our salty tears and perspiration, as well as the chemical composition of amnionic and other body fluids, bear a striking resemblance to sea water. And now, even though we dwell on land, we begin life in the miniature ocean of our mother's womb where, as the late Rachel Carson noted, we evolve ". . . from gill-breathing inhabitants of a water world to creatures able to live on land."[1]

Is it any wonder that, for many of us, water seems to be our natural habitat? Perhaps dim remembrance of eons past, or a desire to again experience the soothing weightlessness we found in our mother's womb, accounts for the proliferation of swimming pools that dot America's landscape like shimmering

[1]Rachel Carson, *The Sea Around Us*. New York: New American Library, 1961, p. 29.

3

turquoise confetti.[2] Whatever the reason for the eternal fascination with our water world, it remains a respite for our gravity-heavy bodies and brings endless pleasure for all those who venture into it.

Why Exercise in the Water?

The first and most obvious reason is the one my students give—"It's such fun!" And right they are. But there are other, more practical reasons why exercise in the water is so special.

To begin with, water is an elastic medium nearly eight hundred times more viscous than air. When in it, you are virtually free of gravity and the stress it produces on your skeletal, respiratory, digestive, and circulatory mechanisms—in other words, on your entire body. Because the spine is in a tenuous vertical position, gravity's compressive force throughout life tends to exaggerate its normal curves, perhaps making you stooped or even sway-backed. In addition to its effect on posture, breathing and internal organ functions are similarly affected by gravity. For instance, the weight of the chest must be lifted with each breath and held up against gravity's continual pull which, over time, acts to force the ribs and internal organs downward, thus compressing the heart, lungs, and abdominal organs.

In a similar way, gravity also affects circulation by hindering the return flow of blood to the heart. Consequently, fluids can accumulate in the lower extremities, causing edema and exacerbating varicose veins. Happily, though, immersion in water has the opposite effect. Just "marinating" in neck-deep water actually stimulates circulation to the extent that cardiac output (the amount of blood the heart pumps through each ventricle every minute) is increased on an average of 32%.[3] Of course, the benefits to the circulation are even greater when you add body movement and the stimulating massaging effect of the water on muscles and peripheral blood vessels. Moreover, the boost immersion gives the circulation may actually help the

[2]Estimates prepared by Hoffman Publications of Fort Lauderdale, Florida, indicate that we are never far from a swimming pool. As of January 1, 1983, there were well over four million pools in the United States, exclusive of the countless three to four foot deep, portable above-ground pools purchased mainly for youngsters, but suitable for many Aquacises.

[3]M. Arborelius, Jr. and others. "Hemodynamic Changes in Man During Immersion with the Head Above Water." *Aerospace Medicine*, Vol. 43, No. 6:592–598, June 1972.

heart recover more quickly from exertion because it isn't working against the force of gravity.

When you stand in water at chest level, your body is nearly weightless, yet the water's gentle support enables you to move your arms or legs slowly with very little effort—an invaluable benefit to people who must keep their exercise on the mild side. On the other hand, the same "thickness," or resistance, that supports you during slow movements also resists your fast, forceful ones. You can prove this to yourself by standing in chest-deep water and swinging your arms in any direction under the surface.[4] Notice how markedly the resistance increases the faster you try to move your limbs. In fact, after a few warm-up moves, you can reach the point where maximum speed is attained and then the resistance increases in relation to the force applied by the muscles. In other words, the greater your speed, force, and range of motion, the greater the water's counterforce. In time, as you gradually increase the intensity of these components, you also will increase your strength, endurance, and flexibility. Furthermore, the water's elasticity accommodates to variations in force or speed of movement at different joint angles, thus providing a constantly changing resistance. As a result, you can apply maximum force throughout the entire arc of motion without undue stress to your joints. This safety factor is another advantage, since the major drawback of land exercise is that it aggravates orthopedic problems. Presumably the reason many students with joint problems report increases in muscular strength and joint mobility, along with decreases in joint pain, is due to this "effort without stress" concept. And, thanks to the water's resistance in every direction of motion, your muscles can work concentrically to help you develop a strong, supple body without carry-over muscle soreness.

But there's more. Because of the water's buoyancy, gravity-defying feats that are difficult, unsafe, or even impossible on land can be accomplished easily. For instance, you can hop, leap, and jump with lightness and joyous freedom.[5] Jogging in the water, unlike jogging on land, allows you to land softly, thereby cushioning your weight-bearing joints and internal organs against the jarring effects of ballistic impact. Moreover, the water's resistance decreases acceleration, and the chance of sustaining any of the momentum injuries associated with land activities is virtually eliminated. In fact, water is the one environment where you can run, jump, and leap without fear of serious injury or, if you should stumble, float up rather than fall

[4] See "Shape-Up Aquacises."

[5] See the "Walk, Jog, Jump, Hop, and Kick" chapter.

down. Finally, the cool water keeps your body from overheating, a major source of fatigue during vigorous land exercise. So, rather than wasting energy to cope with heat loss, this energy can be used instead to become more fit in the water.

Thus, because of the water's uniqueness, you can safely develop the two major components of body fitness—a strong, flexible skeletal muscle system and an efficient cardiovascular system. Also, by following the suggestions in this book, you will derive such corollary benefits as improved posture, coordination, balance, and agility.

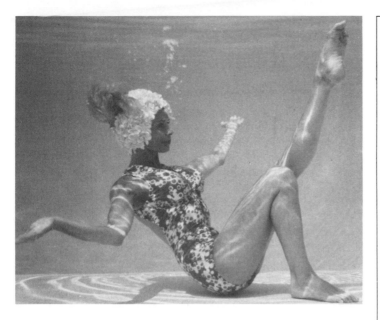

Chapter 2

FROM FIN TO LIMB TO TUCK-IN (IN AND OUT OF THE WATER)

Body Alignment

Scientific findings suggest that our predecessors evolved through the millennia from a water world nearly free of gravity to our gravity-dominated world on land. The first fish-like vertebrates to climb ashore had lungs for breathing air and pectoral fins on which they hobbled about. From them it is thought that all other vertebrates, including ourselves, evolved.

However, unlike other backboned creatures, our upright spine is unsuited to terrestrial life and is prone to anterior/posterior (as seen in profile) distortion from gravitational force. Yet, the antigravity muscles of our legs and trunk, which hold us upright and support our spine, are often weak from inactivity, a condition that contributes to poor posture and a distressing frequency of low back and other chronic physiological problems. Therefore, the purpose of this chapter is to establish guidelines for improving body alignment on land to offset the effects of gravity and for exercise in the water to increase its effectiveness. The primary counterpart to this chapter is the "Shape-Up" group which supplies the know-how for developing the needed strength, endurance, and flexibility of all major muscles, including those important antigravity muscles that help to maintain the spine in alignment.

Our spine has three major curves: lumbar (lower back), thoracic (upper back) and cervical (neck) the degree of which varies among individuals. While there is no one fixed posture for everyone, each person's pelvis, rib cage, and head should be

7

balanced to minimize these curves. Posture of the upper body and head is important. However, the pelvis influences posture more than any other segment of the body. It serves as a base for the flexible portion of the spine, supports the weight of the upper trunk, arms, and head, and transfers it to the legs. If the pelvis is rotated (tipped) forward, the lower back hyperextends, placing considerable stress on the lumbar vertebrae. If it is rotated backward, the curve of the lower back is minimized and the spine is supported to the greatest extent.[6] Any change in the attitude of the pelvis is reflected along the entire length of the spine. Thus, an increased curve of the lower back (sometimes referred to as lumbar lordosis or hollow back) often brings about a rounded upper back, (thoracic kyphosis), round shoulders, and a forward head position. On the other hand, a decrease in the lumbar curve will help to flatten the thoracic curve. Just as the pelvis influences posture of the spine, abdominal muscles most influence pelvic alignment and are, therefore, the key to posture control.

Tuck-In/Stretch Up

Use this procedure to align your spine to minimize its curves. It will contribute to better balance, coordination, economy of movement, and help you use your muscles effectively. Basically, you should think of standing and moving tall. You also may need to

1. Modify the forward curve in your lower back by "tucking-in." Simply TUCK your buttocks under and pull IN your stomach.[7]
2. Align your upper body by lifting your chest (without lifting your shoulders) to a position halfway between a full inspiration and a full expiration.
3. With chin level, flatten the curve at the back of your neck by pressing this area back and stretching upward through the crown of your head.
4. Relax hands, arms, and chest and avoid holding your breath.

[6] The iliac crests (your hipbones) are the anatomic landmarks for pelvic alignment. Forward rotation of the pelvis moves the iliac crests forward; backward rotation moves them back.

[7] Although the word "stomach" properly denotes the principal organ of digestion, it is used in this book to informally describe the abdomen or belly.

When using the Tuck-In/Stretch Up procedure, apply varying degrees of pelvic control according to your needs. For everyday activities, use light control by pulling in your stomach then tucking buttocks under only until you feel a gentle lengthening or "pulling down" through the lower back. Firmer control, especially of the stomach, should be used when doing "Shape-Ups" and similar Aquacises to support the back and align the body for stability against the water's opposing force. Maximum control (maximum backward pelvic tilt) is used in posture-control Aquacises (pp. 110–116) to reinforce the Tuck-in habit, develop stronger abdominal muscles, and help to overcome hollow back.

Developing a kinesthetic awareness of balanced body alignment is fundamental to acquiring better posture. It is the result of frequent reminders to align your spine and repeated efforts to maintain the new position. Ultimately, your reflexes will supplant conscious thought and poised, balanced alignment will occur without direct muscular effort.

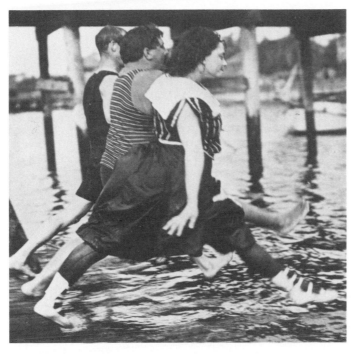

Chapter 3
TAKING THE FIRST STEP

The American Heart Association recommends that sedentary persons contemplating an exercise regimen start with a thorough physical examination. This evaluation should include an examination of the muscles and joints, cardiovascular system, blood pressure, a blood test for cholesterol and triglyceride levels, and a resting electrocardiogram. Also, the AHA recommends an exercise stress test since 10% of "normal" men over 35 have hidden heart disease. However, all other beginning Aquacisers should get their doctor's approval before undertaking this or any other potentially vigorous exercise program.

Planning which Aquacises to use is fun and easy because nearly any combination you choose will make an effective fitness session. Three sample programs are included in the chapter on "Planning Your Water Workouts." When Aquacising, start with light workloads then gradually increase the number of times you repeat the movement as well as the frequency, duration, and intensity of your sessions. Move through your Aquacises with sufficient vigor to feel comfortably tired but not exhausted. However, as your exercise capacity builds, work close to your maximum level during subsequent sessions. Progression should be gradual and based on your adaptation to the workload. This adaptation can be measured by your acquired feeling of energy expenditure (perception of exertion, p. 207), your exercise heart rate (p. 208), and your recovery time after exertion (better conditioning means quicker recovery). To increase your workload and progress to higher fitness levels, incorporate the following four components into your program, *one component at a time:*

REPETITIONS: When you first select the number of times to repeat an Aquacise or the distance or time to kick, walk, jog, or do similar movements, you establish the baseline for measuring your progress as you adapt anatomically and physiologically to the workload. As your exercise tolerance improves, increase the number of repetitions until you can do the maximum number suggested for the Aquacise you are using.

INTENSITY: During your sessions, you can vary the intensity of your effort from easy to hard by adjusting the speed, force, and range (scope) of your movements. For example, for the lightest workloads and heart rates, do Shape-Up and Paddle Aquacises with your working limb completely relaxed (leg/foot or arm/hand). Use only enough force for the limb to drift through the water. For heavier workloads, stretch the working limb to keep the muscles taut and push it forcefully through the water using a full range of motion. Later, increase the speed. At first, you can do Beach Ball Aquacises and Aquabatics with reduced speed and range of motion, then gradually use faster tempos, increased force, and a greater range of motion. When doing other movements such as walking, jogging, and side stepping, start by covering only small distances with each step and, when jumping, use a gentle bobbing action. To intensify these movements, lift the knees high when jogging, cover more distance with every jogging and walking step, and jump higher. Later, increase the tempo so that you are moving faster as well as farther. Use the same idea with swimming kicks—shorter distances in the beginning, longer, faster ones as tolerance increases.

DURATION: In a sea shell, all you need to do initially is keep busy for 15 to 20 minutes (after a brief warm up). In time, try to work up until you can sustain your activity for 30 to 45 minutes. You can do this by repeating your favorite Aquacises, adding new ones to your program, or repeating your program two or three times consecutively.

FREQUENCY: Aquacise a minimum of three days each week and, if time permits, work up to five or six times. In this case, alternate easy and hard days.

Apart from these four basic components, perform your sessions by moving rhythmically and, if possible, continuously. If you must stop, keep it brief. Better yet, learn to pace yourself by slowing down or reducing the force or repetitions to avoid overexertion. Or, change to an Aquacise that uses different muscles. Also, as other alternatives between more vigorous movements, walk slowly through the water while stretching your arms overhead and breathing deeply, or breathe and bob several times.

During your sessions, always remember to:

1. Avoid holding your breath and, after each set of Aquacises, inhale and exhale completely before moving to the next.
2. Relax shoulder and neck muscles.
3. Pull in your stomach and align your body to stand and move tall.
4. Go easy during the first few movements of any Aquacise before using maximum stretch, force, or speed.

Sometimes it takes several sessions before a movement begins to "click." Also, it may take several sessions to develop your balance and stability in vertical positions. Water above chest level (shallower for many people) affects your balance, stability, and traction by diminishing the speed and force of your movements. Therefore, experiment with various water depths (from waist-to-chest-deep) until you find one that permits the greatest stability, force, and range of motion for the Aquacise you are using. Two helpful guidelines: If you can't keep your feet firmly on the pool floor during standing movements, or if you have minimal traction during walking or running movements, the water level is too deep.

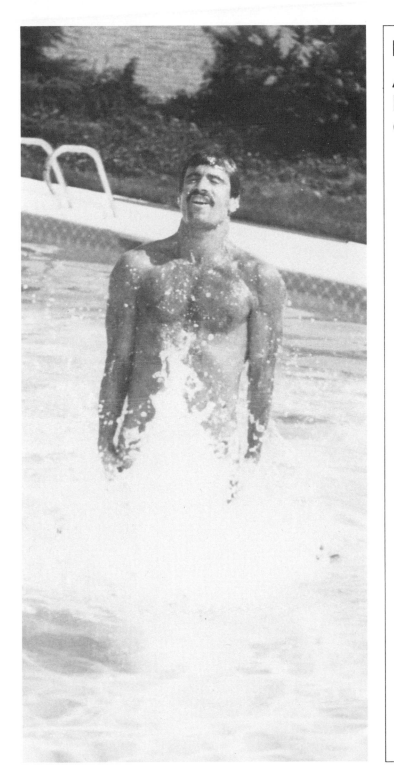

Part II
AQUACISES®
FOR BASIC
CONDITIONING

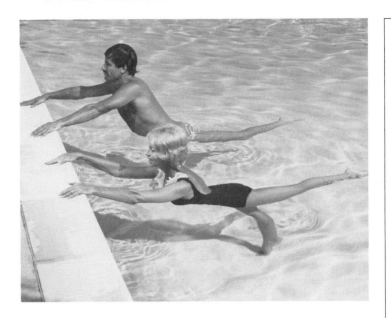

Introduction

Shape-Ups are shallow-water Aquacises that involve large, sweeping arm and leg movements and are done at varying energy levels depending on the range of motion, speed, and force used. Accordingly, they are adaptable both to individuals limited to relatively light workload/heart rates and to apparently healthy individuals who can work up gradually to higher levels. (Page 12 tells how to adjust your workload.) These Shape-Up movements were developed specifically to increase the strength, tone, endurance, and flexibility of the skeletal muscles and, as suggested on pages 208, also to improve cardiovascular efficiency.

Representative movements from each group were tested by the Human Performance Laboratory at Penn State University, using telemetered heart rates which were recorded on an electrocardiograph. Testing concluded that, "The level of exertion may range from a relatively light workload with an average heart rate between 110 and 120 to a much heavier workload with heart rates reaching a person's maximal rate. This variation of work intensity is readily apparent to an observer and may be monitored either by the exercise leader or the exercising individual."

Shape-Ups are divided into the following three categories which correspond to the areas of the body most actively involved in the movements. Include them in your regular swimming regimen or build your fitness sessions around them

17

and Aquacises in the "Walk, Jog, Jump, Hop, and Kick" group as suggested in "Planning Your Water Workouts, Program A."

UPPER LIMBS: This category is comprised of arm movements involving the shoulder girdle and shoulder joint to benefit muscles of the arms and upper trunk (shoulders, chest, and upper back).

TRUNK: These are primarily movements of the trunk (rib cage and pelvic girdle) which affect muscles of the waist, stomach, and back. These movements also involve upper or lower limbs and, thus, benefit those areas as well.

LOWER LIMBS: Most of the Aquacises in this group consist of leg movements emanating from the hip joint and thereby involve muscles of the hips, thighs, and buttocks. For movements that actively involve the lower legs and feet, see the "Walk, Jog, Jump, Hop, and Kick" chapter.

When you perform Shape-Up Aquacises, your muscles will work in a different and most effective way—one not usually experienced with conventional land exercise. To illustrate, let's compare a sequence of muscle contractions occurring during a body movement on land, then during the same movement in the water.

On land, the muscles most involved in lifting a part of the body against the force of gravity shorten or contract concentrically. Then, the same muscle fibers lengthen, or contract eccentrically, to return the part to its starting position (SP). This controlled lengthening prevents the part from falling with the force of gravity. For example, hold onto a stable object and stand on one foot. Now, lift the other leg forward, then lower it to the SP. During the lifting phase, the hip flexors (the muscles at the front of your hip and thigh) contract concentrically to lift your leg against gravity. On the downward phase, they contract eccentrically to control your leg's descent.

In the water, the muscles most involved in lifting the leg forward forcefully (otherwise, your leg tends to float up) also shorten or contract concentrically. However, in the water this action is not followed by an eccentric contraction of those muscles, but by a concentric contraction of the opposing muscle group. In other words, your hip extensors (the muscles at the back of your thigh and hip) contract concentrically to pull your leg down to the SP. This is an advantage because one group of muscles can rest while the opposing group works.

This concept of reciprocal concentric exercise is built into every Shape-Up and Paddle Aquacise. Research has shown that concentric exercise is especially effective in increasing muscular strength. Moreover, it produces little or no residual muscle soreness, even after vigorous beginning workouts. With reciprocal concentric exercise, muscular fitness can be increased in every direction of motion to help the body develop symmetrically.

Upper Limb Shape-Ups

Although swimming is widely recognized as an all-around conditioner, the simple truth is that many people don't swim well enough, or long enough, to realize its benefits. On the other hand, even competent swimmers often find the pool too crowded, the water irritating to the eyes, or lap swimming monotonous.

In this section, I will show you Upper Limb Shape-Ups—a series of alternative arm movements that require no special skills and can be done while standing in waist-to-chest-deep water. (There is always a small space, even in a crowded pool, to do your favorites.) These movements also provide the variety and range of motion missing in swimming strokes. When performed against the water's resistance, Upper Limb Shape-Ups will firm and strengthen the arms, shoulders, upper back, and the supporting muscles of the breasts. Also, they will improve your posture and help you to breathe freely and easily by increasing shoulder and chest flexibility. Even the muscles of your hands and wrists will be strengthened as your fingers work to maintain their extended position against the water's resistance. For added variety, the "Paddle Aquacises" chapter provides more upper limb movements that are done with hand paddles. These Paddle Aquacises are an effective extension of this chapter because they can be used during many of the movements. Those that are particularly appropriate are marked with the symbol (P).

Upper Limb Shape Ups

BOOBY (p. 21)
Basic Movement
Twist and Clap
Hips Back—Hips Forward
One Leg Forward
One Leg Back
Swing Across
Slow 'n Fast
Swing Around—Clap Down

PELICAN (p. 22)
Basic Movement
Double Plunge
Side Plunge

ANEMONE (p. 23)
Basic Movement
Kick Back
Kick Front—Back, Arms in Unison
Kick Front—Back, Arms in Opposition

JACKNIFE FISH (p. 24)
Basic Movement
Jacknife 'n Swing
Stretch Out 'n Swing
Cross Arms and Legs

PUFFIN (p. 25)
Basic Movement
Extend 'n Fly
Float 'n Fly

BUTTERFLYFISH (p. 26)
Basic Movement
Knees Up and Touch
Jump and Touch

MARLIN (p. 26)
Basic Movement
Add a Twist
Clap 'n Fling

OARFISH (p. 27)
Basic and Reverse Movements
Body Slant
One Up
Two Up
Head Up
Tummy Down

SUNSTAR (p. 28)
Use Oarfish to move across pool
Knees Up
Feet Forward
Feet Down
V-Split Low
V-Split High
Frog Knees
Scissors Split

HUMBUG (p. 29)
Basic Movement
Sweep Away

SPOONBILL (p. 30)
Basic Movement

PENGUIN (p. 30)
Basic Movement
One Leg Back
Add a twist
Double Swing
Double Swing with Extra Stretch
Surface Swing

HYDRA (p. 31)
Basic Movement
Double Circle
Jump 'n Circle
Combination
Circle in Unison

WATER BEAR (p. 32)
Hug Yourself
Hug One Knee
Hug Both Knees
Hugh One Thigh
Hug Both Thighs

SAND DOLLAR (p. 33)
Basic Movement
One Leg Back
One Leg Forward
Two Plus One
Circle Side, Hands Clenched
Circle Side, Hands Relaxed

"SMART" SMELT (p. 34)
Basic Movement
Some Choices

Unless advised otherwise, (1) start with 10 repetitions of each of your chosen Upper Limb Shape-Ups and work up to 30, and (2) keep fingers together for maximum water resistance.

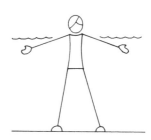

FIGURE 4-1

BOOBY (P)

Firms arms, upper body, and shoulders; increases flexibility in shoulders and chest. Most variations trim the waist and strengthen the stomach.

GET SET: Stand in **water at shoulder level** with feet apart side to side or front to back. Hold arms sideward and back as far as possible, hands just under the surface, palms facing forward (Fig. 4-1). Palms remain in this fixed position throughout the movements. Pull in your stomach.

GO: Sweep arms forward and clap hands In front, then sweep them back to the start. Keep elbows and fingers straight, hands under the surface of the water.

VARIATIONS:

Twist and Clap. Begin with arms In the **Get Set** position, feet apart to the side. Now, twist right at the waist so that shoulders face right. Hold the twist while you swing arms forward to clap hands (Fig. 4-2), then swing arms back. Next, twist all the way to the left so that shoulders face left, then clap again. As you twist, keep hands just under the surface, arms constantly sideward (as if an imaginary pole were stretched across your shoulders from fingertip to fingertip). Most importantly, pull in your stomach.

Hips Back—Hips Forward. Thrust your hips back and bend forward as you swing arms forward (Fig. 4-3); then thrust hips forward as you move arms back (Fig. 4-4). Keep stomach pulled in.

One Leg Forward. Perform **Booby** with one leg raised to the front. As arms move forward, reach toward your toes (Fig. 4-5). As arms move back, lean back slightly and stretch leg forward (Fig. 4-6). Keep toes at the surface, leg muscles taut, foot extended (toes pointed). Repeat several times then change to the opposite leg.

One Leg Back. Perform **Booby** with trunk forward, one leg raised high to the back. For balance, bend supporting knee slightly

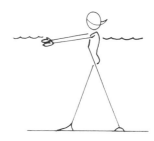

FIGURE 4-2

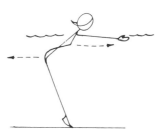

FIGURE 4-3

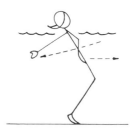

FIGURE 4-4

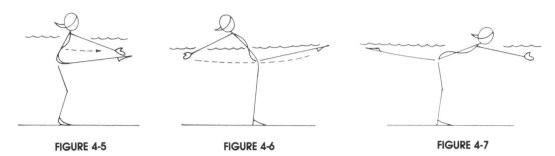

FIGURE 4-5   FIGURE 4-6   FIGURE 4-7

and stretch the back leg with buttocks muscle taut. When arms move forward, stretch from fingertips to toes (Fig. 4-7); when arms move back, maintain forward-trunk position. Repeat several times then change to the opposite leg.

Swing Across. Perform **Booby** but omit clapping hands. Instead, cross one arm over the other—first right over left, then left over right, etc., keeping elbows straight.

Slow 'n Fast. Alternate four slow **Boobys** using your full range of motion, with eight short, fast ones. Repeat the sequence two or more times.

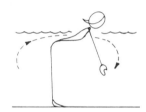

FIGURE 4-8

Swing Around—Clap Down. Instead of swinging arms horizontally, swing them in an arc diagonally down in front and clap hands (Fig. 4-8). Then, reverse the motion swinging arms around to the side and clap down behind your back (Fig. 4-9). Lean forward as arms move down in front; lean back as they move down in back.

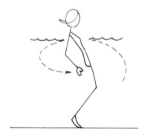

FIGURE 4-9

PELICAN

Vigorous exercise for arms and entire trunk

GET SET: Stand with your right foot forward, left foot back. Put your left hand on your hip and hold your right arm forward above shoulder level. Curl fingers to make a fist (Fig. 4-10).

GO: Plunge your right arm down into the water, past your leg and up to the back. (Turn head and shoulders to watch hand emerge, Fig. 4-11.) Reverse the motion, plunging hand down and forward to the SP. Bend knees as arm moves down; straighten them as arm moves up. After several repetitions, reverse foot position and do **Pelican** with the left arm.

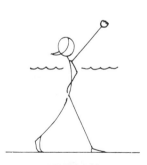

FIGURE 4-10

VARIATIONS:

Double Plunge. Repeat the basic movement but swing arms simultaneously. Start with arms high to the front and finish with them above the surface at each side, stretched back as far as possible (Fig. 4-12). Keep head and shoulders facing forward.

Side Plunge. This time stand with feet apart to the side and swing your arm from side to side. Keep shoulders facing forward (Fig. 4-13) and change to the other arm after several repetitions.

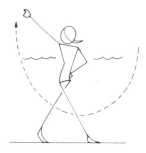

FIGURE 4-11

ANEMONE (P)

Provides Booby benefits; also strengthens and firms muscles of lower trunk and thighs

GET SET: Stand with feet together in **chest-deep water.** Hold your arms sideward, hands just under the surface, with palms facing forward.

GO: Use the **Booby** arm movement. However, as arms move forward, kick one leg forward (Fig. 4-14). As arms swing back, press leg down to the start and stand upright. Be sure to kick high to bring your toes to the surface, but keep knee straight and foot extended. Repeat, alternating legs.

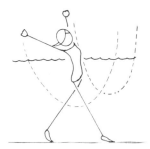

FIGURE 4-12

VARIATIONS:

Kick Back. This time, kick your leg up to the back as you swing arms forward (Fig. 4-15). Press leg down to the start and stand upright as you move arms back. As arms move forward, lean forward slightly to bring leg high and stretch from fingers to toes. Keep stomach pulled in. Alternate legs.

Kick Front—Back, Arms in Unison. Kick your leg back and forth. Kick it forward as arms move forward (Fig. 4-14); then press it

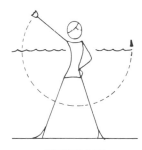

FIGURE 4-13

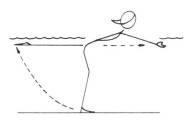

FIGURE 4-15

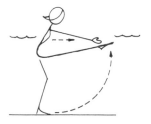

FIGURE 4-14

down and up to the back as arms move back (Fig. 4-16). Kick high with leg stretched, stomach pulled in. After several repetitions, change to the other leg.

Kick Front—Back, Arms in Opposition. This time swing arms back as leg moves forward (Fig. 4-17); then swing arms forward as leg moves back (Fig. 4-18). Repeat several times before changing to the opposite leg.

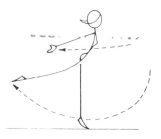

FIGURE 4-16

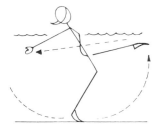

FIGURE 4-17

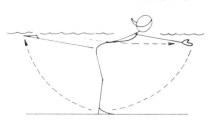

FIGURE 4-18

JACKNIFE FISH (P)

Firms and trims arms, thighs, and trunk; increases flexibility in hips and shoulders

GET SET: In **chest-deep water,** stand on your toes with feet wide apart side to side. Hold arms sideward, hands just under the surface, palms tilted slightly forward, Pull in your stomach; stretch and tense your legs.

GO: Move into a tight jacknife position by swinging your legs together in front. At the same time, swing your arms forward and reach toward your toes (Figs. 4-19 and 4-20). Immediately reverse palm position (turn them to face back) and swing arms and legs back to the start, separating legs wide as you press them sideward and down. Swing arms close to the surface and lift legs high in front, leg muscles always taut, feet extended. Note that the forward-backward arm motion with palms tilted in the direction of motion keeps your head above the surface.

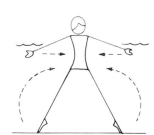

FIGURE 4-19

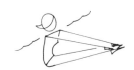

FIGURE 4-20

VARIATIONS:

Jacknife 'n Swing. Use the **Jacknife Fish** arm motion but, instead of returning legs to the SP each time, maintain the sharp angle at the hips while you briskly open-close legs and arms. Keep stomach in, back erect. Repeat 15 or more times or try several sequences of 8 basic **Jacknife Fish** alternated with 8 of this variation.

Stretch Out 'n Swing. Lie front down and spread-eagled on the surface with your head up (Fig. 4-21). Tighten buttocks, stretch legs, and lift heels. Now, press legs together as you swing arms forward (Fig. 4-22) then reverse the motion to the start. Swing briskly with your heels and hands close to the surface. For a more vigorous arm motion, pull arms all the way back to your sides. And, like other **Jacknife Fish** movements, tilt your palms in the direction of motion.

Cross Arms and Legs. Instead of stopping the forward motion as arms and legs come together during the basic **Jacknife Fish** and variations, try crossing them, right over left, then left over right, etc.

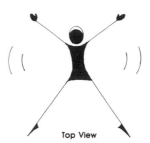

FIGURE 4-21

PUFFIN

Flap your arms like the Puffin which flies both under the water and in the air. You won't go anywhere, but the arm action plus the water's resistance will firm and strengthen muscles of the arms and upper body. In addition, the variations strengthen muscles of the back and buttocks.

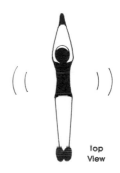

FIGURE 4-22

GET SET: Stand in **chest-deep water** with feet either together or apart side to side. Hold arms sideward, hands just under the surface, palms down. Bend forward slightly.

GO: Flap your arms with fingers, wrists, and elbows completely relaxed. Cut a wide swath through the water, swinging arms straight down and touching hands together before swinging arms up to the surface.

VARIATIONS:

Extend 'n Fly. After doing the basic **Puffin,** try it with one leg extended high to the back. Lean forward and try to bring heel up to surface level (Fig. 4-23). Stretch and tense your leg and repeat the arm motion several times before changing to the opposite leg. After this and other movements that hyperextend the lumbar area (arch your back), stand upright and clasp one knee to your chest. Hold the position briefly, then change to the other leg. This releases tension in lower back muscles sometimes caused by hyperextension.

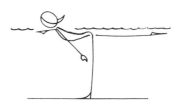

FIGURE 4-23

Float 'n Fly. This time do the arm motion with your body floating front down on the surface, head up, legs together (Fig. 4-24) or

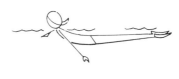

FIGURE 4-24

apart in a wide V-split. Stretch legs, tighten buttocks, and lift heels with feet extended. If pool steps are available, they may be used to support your feet.

BUTTERFLYFISH (P)

Firms arms, shoulders, and upper body

GET SET: Stand with feet together in **chest-to-shoulder-deep water.** Hold arms sideward, hands just under the surface, palms down.

GO: Press your arms down to your sides, then lift them up to the start. Pump arms vigorously, keeping elbows and fingers straight, hands under the surface (Fig. 4-25). For a bouncy effect, keep feet on the floor and bend knees as arms move up; straighten knees as arms move down.

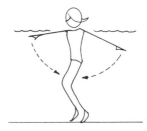

FIGURE 4-25

VARIATIONS:

Knees Up and Touch. Perform the basic movement but, as arms move down, lift your knees and touch fingertips to ankles (Fig. 4-26). Reverse the motion to return to the start. You can perform this variation during each, or every other, downward arm motion.

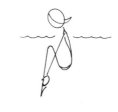

Jump and Touch. Perform the previous variation while moving forward around the shallow end of the pool. Just give a little forward jump as you lift your knees.

FIGURE 4-26

MARLIN

Strengthens arms, shoulders, and upper body. Stretches shoulders and chest. Second variation adds waist exercise.

GET SET: Stand in **lower-chest-deep water** with your feet apart side to side. With your fingers curled into fists, extend arms low in front, thumbs touching.

GO: Swing one arm forward and overhead as you swing the other back (Fig. 4-27). Reverse the motion, alternating arms. After several warm-up moves, fling arms vigorously. Keep elbows straight and move arms back as far as possible.

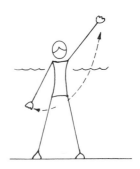

FIGURE 4-27

VARIATIONS:

Clap 'n Fling. For more water resistance, perform **Marlin** with fingers straight then brush palms together as they move past the start.

Add a Twist. Perform **Marlin** as instructed, but turn head and shoulders to watch the hand moving to the back; turn front as arm swings down and to the SP. Next, repeat the action in the opposite direction.

OARFISH (P)

Firms and strengthens arms, shoulders, and upper body

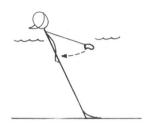

GET SET: Stand with **water at lower-chest level,** feet apart front to back. Extend arms forward at the surface, palms down, thumbs touching. This gets you ready for the **Basic** and **Reverse Oarfish** arm movements.

GO: In a motion resembling the breast stroke, forcefully pull your arms back through the water, turning palms outward slightly to increase resistance. Bend elbows to bring hands around to the front, then straighten arms forward to the SP.
    To reverse the motion, bend elbows and slide hands toward you, all the way back past your sides. Straighten elbows and turn palms to face forward so that you're ready to forcefully scoop arms forward. For both the basic and reverse movements, increase chest and shoulder flexibility by always pulling arms back past level of shoulders. Practice the above movements separately, then repeat several sequences of eight **Basic Oarfish** alternating with eight **Reverse Oarfish**.

FIGURE 4-28

VARIATIONS:

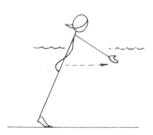

FIGURE 4-29

Body Slant. Peform the basic arm movement while you lean backward (Fig. 4-28). Next, perform the reverse motion while leaning forward (Fig. 4-29). For proper position, lean back or forward from the ankles, heels pressed toward the floor, body straight and stiff. Maintain this angle by holding a firm Tuck-in and stroking continuously. Stroke eight or more times in each position and repeat the sequence several times.

One Up. Perform the basic arm movement while facing the wall with the sole of one foot braced high on the wall, knee straight (Fig. 4-30). After several repetitions, change to the other leg. This version, as well as the next, will increase flexibility in your back and the back of your legs.

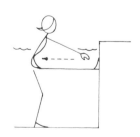

FIGURE 4-30

Two Up. Perform the basic arm movement at a brisk pace with the soles of both feet flat against the wall, knees straight. Brace your feet high on the wall, back erect, stomach pulled in (Fig. 4-31). As with all **Oarfish** movements, stretch arms forward and touch thumbs together each time. If your hamstring muscles are too tight to bring feet into position, at first do this variation with knees bent and only your toes against the wall.

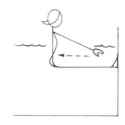

FIGURE 4-31

Head Up. Use the reverse arm movement while sitting in the water with your back toward the wall. Place the soles of your feet against the wall with heels close to buttocks. Lean forward slightly so that hands clear the wall (Fig. 4-32). Keep feet in place, back straight.

Tummy Down. Use the reverse arm motion while floating on your front, head up, and with the soles of your feet flat against the wall (Fig. 4-33). Perform at a brisk pace and scoop arms forward forcefully to keep feet in place.

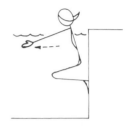

FIGURE 4-32

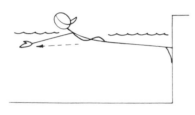

FIGURE 4-33

SUNSTAR (P)

Firms arms, upper trunk, and abdomen

GET SET: Stand in **chest-deep water,** back erect, stomach pulled in. Extend arms forward at the surface, palms down, thumbs together.

GO: Use the **Basic** and **Reverse Oarfish** arm movements to cruise forward or backward around the pool with your legs in the various positions listed below. Try them all because each version offers a new challenge to body control and balance. As you move along, keep back erect, stomach in.

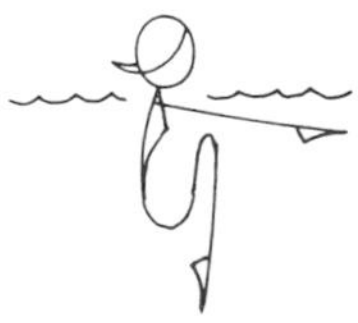

Knees Up. Tuck your knees toward your chest (Fig. 4-34).

Feet Forward. Stretch your legs forward at right angles to your body—legs together, knees straight, and feet extended (Fig.

FIGURE 4-34

4-35). Even better, lift legs higher to bring toes to the surface, but keep your back erect.

Feet Down. In **chin-deep water,** extend your legs straight down, feet together. Tuck-in tightly, stretch your legs, and extend your feet (Fig. 4-36).

V-Split Low. Separate your legs to the side in a wide V-split. Stretch and tense legs and extend feet (Fig. 4-37).

V-Split High. Separate legs to the side in a wide V-split, legs forward at right angles to your body. Stretch and tense legs, extend feet (Fig. 4-38).

Frog Knees. With the soles of your feet together, bend your knees, pressing them outward in "frog" fashion.

Scissors Split. Separate legs front to back in a wide scissors split. Periodically reverse their position to bring the opposite leg forward. Lift your chest, stretch and tense legs, and extend feet (Fig. 4-39).

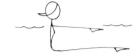

FIGURE 4-35

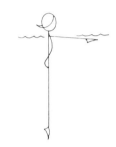

FIGURE 4-36

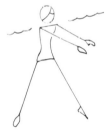

FIGURE 4-37

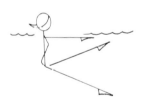

FIGURE 4-38

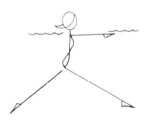

FIGURE 4-39

HUMBUG (P)

Firms arms and all muscles of the trunk

GET SET: Stand in **chest-deep water** with feet apart side to side, hands on hips. Pull in your stomach.

GO: Sweep arms forward in wide arcs, one arm at a time. First, reach the right arm back; sweep it out to the side and across in front to the left (Fig. 4-40). Then bend elbow and pull hand back to hip. Next, use the same action with the left arm. Move each arm through the greatest arc possible, twisting at the

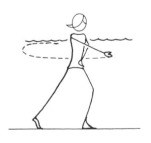

FIGURE 4-40

waist to extend its range. As arm sweeps across, push palm against the water, fingers straight, hand just under the surface. (It's appropriate to hum during this Aquacise.)

VARIATION:

Sweep Away. Reverse the sweep across motion and push the water away with the back of your hand and arm. First, reach right arm across to the left, straightening elbow as you reach. Now, sweep arm around to the right as far as possible (Fig. 4-41) and put hand on hip. Next, use the same action with the left arm, sweeping it to the left.

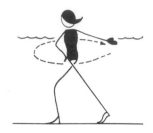

FIGURE 4-41

SPOONBILL (P)

Firms arms, upper body, and waist; increases flexibility of shoulders and chest

GET SET: Stand facing the wall, arms' length away, with your feet apart side to side. Bend forward from the hips until the **water is at shoulder level.** Hold the ledge with the right hand and extend your left arm straight down.

GO: Swing left arm up to the surface at the right side, then swing it down past vertical and up to the surface at the left. Or, you can enlarge the motion and lift your arm out of the water at each side (Fig. 4-42). After several repetitions, change to the left arm. Keep back straight and stomach pulled in.

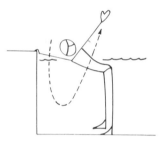

FIGURE 4-42

PENGUIN (P)

Firms arms, shoulders, and upper body. The first variation also strengthens lower back and buttocks while the second trims the waist.

GET SET: Stand in **water at shoulder level** with feet apart front to back. Hold your right arm forward just beneath the surface, palm down, and your left arm back, palm facing up (Fig. 4-43).

GO: Exchange the position of your arms. As the right arm presses down and back, press the left arm down and forward. Swing arms forcefully with elbows and fingers straight. Be sure to swing arms *down* past your legs before lifting them to the surface at the end of each motion.

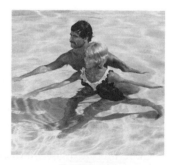

FIGURE 4-43

VARIATIONS:

One Leg Back. Perform **Penguin** with one leg raised high to the back. Keep leg stretched and tensed, buttocks taut, foot extended (Fig. 4-44). As arms move to the front, reach forward to maximum stretch. After several repetitions change to the other leg.

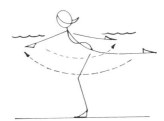

FIGURE 4-44

Add a Twist. Stand with feet apart side to side. Perform the basic movement, but twist to the right as your left arm moves forward (Fig. 4-45) then press arms down to your sides. Next, twist left as your right arm moves forward.

Double Swing. Swing arms down and up as in the basic movement, but in the same direction simultaneously.

Double Swing with Extra Stretch. Also try **Double Swing** with one leg raised high to the front. First, swing arms forward and reach toward toes (Fig. 4-46); then swing arms back as you lean back and stretch your leg forward as if you were being pulled by the toes (Fig. 4-47). After several repetitions, repeat with the opposite leg forward.

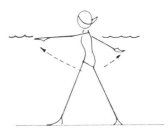

FIGURE 4-45

Surface Swing. Instead of the up-down arm motion, swing arms horizontally, hands vertical and just under the surface, thumbs uppermost. Start with feet apart side to side, right arm forward, left arm back. Now, swing right arm back as you swing the left arm forward; then reverse the motion, swinging arms around to the left. Keep shoulders facing front, palms in a fixed position. Swing arms back as far as possible each time.

HYDRA

Firms arms and all muscles of the trunk

GET SET: Stand with feet apart side to side in **waist-to-chest-deep water.** Put your right hand on your hip and extend your left arm sideward at shoulder level, fingers straight, palm facing down.

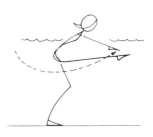

FIGURE 4-46

GO: With elbow straight, swing your left arm in a large circle in front (Fig. 4-48). First, swing it down and across in front, then overhead and out to the SP. As your hand enters the water, plunge it vigorously downward and bend your knees. As it swings upward, straighten knees and fling water high into the air. (People with shoulder or elbow problems can reduce the water's resistance by making fists with their hands.) Periodically (1) circle in the opposite direction and (2) repeat with the right arm.

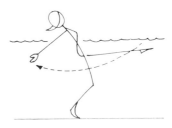

FIGURE 4-47

VARIATIONS:

Double Circle. Now, circle arms simultaneously. Start by standing on the balls of your feet and extend arms sideward at shoulder level, fingers straight or curled into fists. Tuck-in. Next, vigorously swing arms down in front, crossing one over the other (Fig. 4-49) or bring palms together instead. Follow through by lifting arms overhead and flinging water high into the air; then separate arms out to the side SP (Fig. 4-50). (In other words, each arm makes a big circle.) Bend knees as arms move down; straighten them and stretch as arms move up.

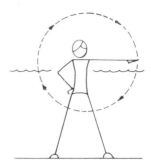

FIGURE 4-48

Jump 'n Circle. Use the **Double Circle** movement and jump twice each time your arms circle. Jump once as you plunge arms down, then jump again as you swing them up.

Combination. Perform several repetitions of the basic movement with each arm followed by several **Double Circles.** Repeat the sequence several times, sometimes reversing the direction of the circles.

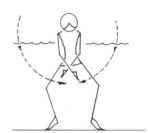

FIGURE 4-49

Circle in Unison. This time start with both arms over to the left above the surface about shoulder width apart (Fig. 4-51). Now you're ready to circle them simultaneously in the same direction. First, plunge arms down into the water, past the front of your legs, and up to the right; then overhead (fling water into the air) and down to the SP. After several circles, reverse direction.

WATER BEAR (P)

Firms arms and trunk; increases flexibility in chest, shoulders, and back

GET SET: Stand erect with feet together in **chest-deep water,** arms sideward and back as far as possible, elbows straight, hands just under the surface. Turn palms to face forward.

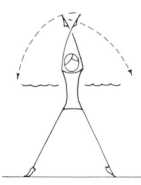

FIGURE 4-50

GO: Use this series of movements separately or in sequence by repeating each several times before moving to the next.

Hug Yourself: Give yourself a big bear hug. Just swing your arms forward and cross them in front of your chest, bending your elbows. Then press them back to the SP.

Hug One Knee. This time swing arms forward as you lift one knee and clasp it close to your chest. Reverse the motion and press arms and leg back to the SP. Repeat, alternating legs.

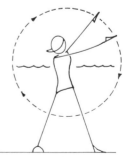

FIGURE 4-51

Hug Both Knees. Now, lift both knees as you swing arms forward and clasp knees close to your chest (Fig. 4-52). Be sure to keep knees together and lift them high. However, don't jump up at the start. Instead, lift your knees and use smooth, forceful arm pressure to keep your head above the surface.

Hug One Thigh. Start with palms down, then lift one knee toward your chest as you press arms straight down and clasp them around your thigh. Stand erect again as you press arms and leg to the SP, then repeat with the left thigh.

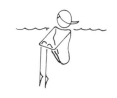

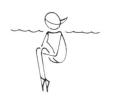

FIGURE 4-52

Hug Both Thighs. Turn palms down, then lift both knees as you press arms down and clasp both thighs (Fig. 4-53). Stand erect again as you press arms and legs to the start. As with **Hug Both Knees,** do not jump up at the start.

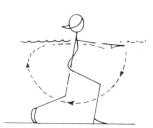

FIGURE 4-53

SAND DOLLAR (P)

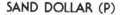

Firms arms and upper trunk; increases flexibility of chest and shoulders. The first three variations add lower trunk and thigh exercise.

GET SET: Stand in **lower-chest-deep water** with feet apart front to back, then bend your knees until the water is at shoulder level. Hold arms forward at the surface, palms down, thumbs together.

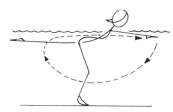

FIGURE 4-54

GO: Rotate your arms in large circles, keeping elbows and fingers straight, hands under the surface. Arms should move through their greatest range of motion, circling down past your legs, far to the back, then through the forward SP (Fig. 4-54). After several repetitions, reverse direction, keeping palms always turned to face direction of motion.

VARIATIONS:

One Leg Back. Circle your arms with one leg lifted up to the back, leg stretched, buttocks taut. Lean forward to bring leg high and lift your chest (Fig. 4-55). After several repetitions, reverse direction then repeat with the opposite leg back.

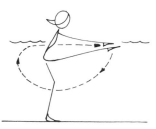

FIGURE 4-55

One Leg Forward. Circle arms with one leg raised forward, toes at the surface. Stretch and tense your leg, extend your foot, and pull in your stomach. As arms move forward, reach toward your toes (Fig. 4-56). After several repetitions, reverse direction, then repeat with the opposite leg forward

FIGURE 4-56

Two Plus One. Stand in **chest-deep water,** one leg raised high in front, hands in the forward SP. Now, circle arms and leg simultaneously, bringing them down, back, then around to the start (Fig. 4-57). Keep both knees straight, working leg stretched. After several repetitions, perform with opposite leg.

Circle Side, Hands Clenched. With arms sideward, hands under the surface, perform a series of small, fast circles with elbows straight, hands clenched into fists. For maximum stretch to chest and shoulders, circle arms back as far as possible, changing direction after every eight circles. For further variation, perform several sequences of eight small, fast circles with hands clenched, followed by four large circles with fingers straight. Then, do it again by circling in the opposite direction.

Circle Side, Hands Relaxed. Start again with arms sideward and perform a series of small, fast circles with fingers and wrists completely relaxed. Circle arms as far back as possible each time, changing direction after every eight circles. Concentrate on relaxing hands while pushing arms forcefully through the water.

Note. If using paddles, omit the last two variations.

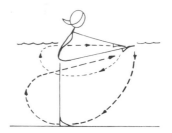

FIGURE 4-57

"SMART" SMELT

Firms arms, shoulders, upper body

GET SET: Stand with feet apart front to back, arms sideward, stomach pulled in. Bend knees to bring the **water level to your shoulders.**

GO: Moving arms in unison, draw imaginary numbers from one to ten (Fig. 4-58). Then, work your way back from ten to one. Make the movements as large as possible, keeping elbows and fingers straight, hands under the surface.

VARIATION:

Some Choices. In addition to numbers only, try writing the alphabet or your name and address.

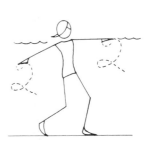

FIGURE 4-58

Trunk Shape-Ups

Have you ever wondered why you've never seen a fish with a flabby stomach? We marvel at their fluid grace, but seldom consider the strong set of trunk muscles that fish use for propulsion. While humans aren't required to use their trunk muscles primarily for locomotion, they should be used naturally in other ways to keep them strong.

Abdominal muscles should be actively employed both in the breathing process and to help maintain an upright posture. Quiet breathing hardly activates them and we nearly always sit and stand hunched over with our stomach slack and our spine curved outward like a cocktail shrimp. When we give in to sedentary living and avoid the vigorous activities that develop and maintain trunk muscle tone, we often end up with poor posture, a protruding stomach, weakened back muscles, and the potential for low-back problems. Therefore, since these conditions concern many of us, this section will stress Aquacises that involve all muscles of the trunk, especially those of the midsection.

Strong abdominals are particularly important since they support the internal organs against the downward force of gravity and are the basic stabilizers of the lumbar area. Similarly, a strong, flexible trunk, which contributes to graceful body movements, is also the best insurance against low-back problems. The most important abdominal muscles span the area from the ribs to the pelvis. They are (1) the rectus abdominis (a thick, fairly slim muscle lying vertically along the front of your belly), (2) the transverse abdominis (lying under the rectus, with fibers running at right angles to it), and (3) the internal and external obliques (lying on top of and at nearly right angles to one another, along the front and side of the abdomen). The abdominals and the erector spinae group (layers of closely knit muscles that extend the length of your back from pelvis to neck on both sides of your spine) form a muscular girdle around your midsection and work in harmony to keep the spinal column aligned.

The trunk itself can move in a variety of ways. However, the degree of possible movement depends on the vertebral bony structure, the shape and thickness of the intervertebral discs, the length and tautness of the ligaments, and the flexibility of the muscles producing the motion. With the lumbar spine as a pivotal support, the trunk can flex, extend, hyperextend, flex laterally, rotate, and flex and extend diagonally. Then too, the pelvis can move independently. It can rotate forward and backward, laterally and, to a lesser extent, from side to side. This group of Trunk Shape-Ups utilizes all of these ranges of motion to actively involve the muscles under discussion.

Trunk Shape-Ups

In addition to the Aquacises in this group, it is worth noting that muscles of the abdominal girdle are involved in nearly every movement we make against the water's resistance. For instance, when performing Shape-Ups for upper or lower limbs, the muscles that connect the pelvis to the rib cage (along with those that join the rib cage to the head) act to stabilize you against the water's counterforce. Moreover, during lower limb movements, they help align the pelvis so that your limb can move freely through its full range of motion. Too, the greater this range, the more vigorously your abdominal girdle muscles are involved.

To enhance the effects of Trunk Shape-Ups, you should develop the habit of pulling in your stomach. Dieting is important too if you are overweight and have to contend with an accumulation of fat around your middle. Remember, whether you call it a promontory, a protuberance, or a pot, a conspicuous stomach is unbecoming and the related low-back problems can be painful!

Unless advised otherwise, start with 10 repetitions of each of your chosen Trunk Shape-Ups and work up to 30.

TRUNKFISH

Strengthens arms and increases strength and flexibility of trunk for a firm, supple body

GET SET: Stand with feet apart side to side in **chest-deep water,** arms forward, hands shoulder-width apart. Turn palms to face one another, hands just under the surface, elbows straight. For greatest resistance, maintain this spacing between hands so that arms and upper body move as a unit.

GO: Repeat any of the following movements six or more times to each side. Better yet, do them all in sequence by repeating each several times before moving onto the next. Get your trunk into the action by bending and twisting at the waist. This adds waist exercise and enables the arms to move through a greater range of motion.

Arms Across. Swing your arms from side to side, moving them as far as possible in each direction (Fig. 4-59).

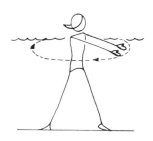

FIGURE 4-59

Arms Across and Down. Swing arms in an arc, moving them across in front, then down toward the back (Fig. 4-60). Reverse direction to the SP at the other side.

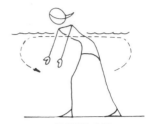

FIGURE 4-60

Arms Down and Up. This time start with arms to one side. Now, swing them down in front of your legs and up to the other side. Continue the pendulum-like motion swinging arms low on the downward phase (Fig. 4-61).

Arms Down—Circle and Up. Again start with arms to one side. First, swing them down, then up across in front and down again in a large circle. Complete the motion by swinging arms up to the other side (Fig. 4-62). Reverse the entire procedure ending with arms in the SP.

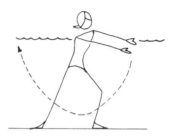

FIGURE 4-61

Arms Low. Bend forward with arms perpendicular to floor. Now, swing them in an arc around to the other side and toward the back (Fig. 4-63). Reverse direction, bringing arms across in front to the other side. Keep hands at a constant level and stomach pulled in.

Single-Handed. Repeat any **Trunkfish** movement using one arm at a time with the other hand resting on your hip.

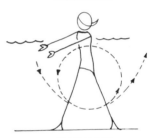

FIGURE 4-62

SAWFISH

Firms arms and trunk, especially the waist

GET SET: Stand in **chest-deep water** with feet apart side to side. Extend arms forward, shoulder-width apart, with hands just under the surface, palms facing right. Pull in your stomach.

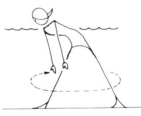

FIGURE 4-63

GO: Lean forward; then in one continuous, sweeping motion, press your hands through the water to the right. (Twist at the waist for maximum stretch, Fig. 4-64.) As you complete this action, bend your elbows and pull your hands to your hips (palm of left hand to the right hip, palm of right hand across in back to the left hip, Fig. 4-65). Next, reverse the entire motion and palm direction, swinging arms across in front and around to the left.

VARIATION:

Swish. Stand with feet apart, hands on your hips. Now twist at the waist, swinging your shoulders quickly from side to side so

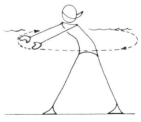

FIGURE 4-64

that your elbows make a swishing sound as they move through the water. Keep your stomach pulled in.

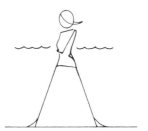

FIGURE 4-65

GRUNION

Firms arms and trunk

GET SET: Stand with feet together in **lower-chest-deep water,** then bend knees to bring the water level to your chest. Hold arms in a fixed, wide V position, hands just under the surface. Tuck-in.

GO: Briskly swing knees from side to side as you pivot on the balls of your feet (Fig. 4-67). For more upper body and arm benefits, swing your arms horizontally, opposite to the direction of your knees.

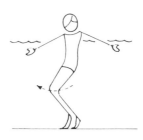

FIGURE 4-66

CROAKER

A fine conditioner for waist and stomach. Also strengthens supporting arm.

GET SET: Stand on your toes in **chest-deep water** with your left side facing the wall, about three feet out. Lean toward the wall on a slant and hold the ledge with your left hand. Extend your right arm sideward, hand in the water. Pull in your stomach and stretch/tense your legs (Fig. 4-68).

GO: In a smooth, continuous motion, tuck up knees as you swing feet up and across in front toward the wall at the left. As feet pass in front, roll to the right hip, then touch feet to the wall (Fig. 4-69). Reverse the motion, pushing feet away from the wall and down to the SP. Keep legs together and use your left arm in push-pull fashion to help change

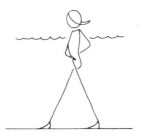

FIGURE 4-67

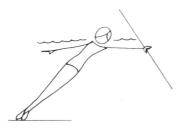

FIGURE 4-68

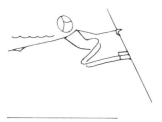

FIGURE 4-69

position. Use the right arm as a stabilizing rudder. To make this movement more vigorous, jump once to lift feet up to the wall, then jump again, pushing your feet away from the wall down to the start. Periodically perform with right side toward the wall.

VARIATIONS:

Tuck 'n Turn. Begin in the slanted SP. Now, as you tuck up your knees, turn to face the wall and touch your toes to the wall in front (Fig. 4-70). Then, push your feet back and down as you turn to the side-slanted SP. After several repetitions, start with right side toward the wall, right hand holding pool rim. To vary, instead of the slanted SP, begin and end in the side-floating position shown in Fig. 4-71.

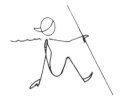

FIGURE 4-70

Extend Sideward. Tuck up knees and touch feet to the wall as suggested in the basic movement. However, instead of the slanted SP, begin and end this variation in the side-floating position shown in Figure 4-71. Legs should be together and stretched, feet extended and close to the surface. After several repetitions, perform on your right side, right hand holding the rim.

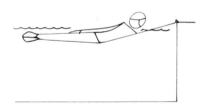

FIGURE 4-71

TURNSTONE

Firms and trims waist, stomach, hips, buttocks, and thighs

GET SET: In **chest-deep water,** stand on the balls of your feet facing the wall about two feet out. Lean forward on a slant and hold the ledge, hands shoulder-width apart. Bend your right knee to the side, foot extended, toes braced against the inside of your left knee (Fig. 4-72).

GO: Moving from the hip joint, briskly swing your knee across in front to the left, then reverse to the SP. In other words,

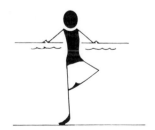

FIGURE 4-72

swing your knee from side to side. At the same time, pivot on your left foot to bring knee as far as possible to each side. Keep stomach in and change legs after several repetitions.

VARIATIONS:

Bubble Up. Starting in the **Get Set** position, swing knee left, then right to the start. Next, straighten knee, lifting toes to the surface at the side, knee cap facing up (Fig. 4-73). Bend knee and repeat the sequence, moving continuously from one position to the next. Lift foot upward smoothly (to feel the stretch in inner thigh) or with a jabbing motion. After several repetitions, change to the left leg.

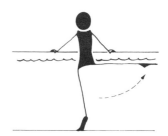

FIGURE 4-73

Snap Back. From the **Get Set** position, swing knee left then right. Next, straighten knee to the back, bending forward slightly (stretch leg up and back, Fig. 4-74). Stand upright again, bending knee to the side SP and repeat the sequence moving continuously from one position to the next. Either extend leg back smoothly or with a jabbing motion. After several repetitions, perform with the left leg.

Side View. Do the basic movement while standing erect with left side facing the wall. Hold the ledge with the left hand and swing your right knee from side to side. After several repetitions, perform with the right side facing the wall and swing your left knee.

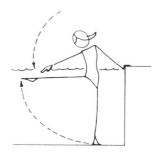

FIGURE 4-74

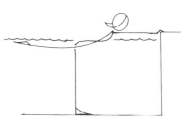

FIGURE 4-75

NAIAD

Firms and stretches the trunk laterally and strengthens the thigh, hip, and buttock of the working leg. The second variation firms/stretches front and back of the trunk.

GET SET: Stand in **waist-to-chest-deep water** with your left side toward the wall, feet together. Hold the ledge with your left hand and raise your right arm overhead. Pull in your stomach.

GO: Kick your right leg to the side as you lower your right arm to reach toward your toes (Fig. 4-75). Press your leg down as you swing right arm overhead and sway to the left, reaching toward the pool deck (Fig. 4-76). Be sure to kick high with leg fully stretched and foot extended. Sway directly to the side without turning your shoulders. After several repetitions, perform with the left leg, right side toward the wall.

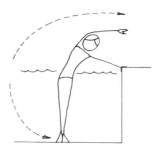

FIGURE 4-76

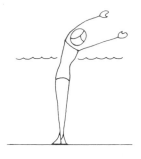

FIGURE 4-77

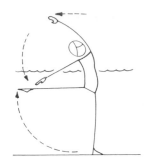

FIGURE 4-78

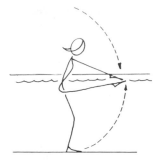

FIGURE 4-79

VARIATIONS:

Stand Free, Sway Side. Perform the basic movement standing away from the wall with both arms overhead (Figs. 4-77 and 4-78).

Sway Forward and Back. Use the basic movement SP, but this time kick your right leg forward as you lower the right arm and reach toward your toes (Fig. 4-79). Next, reverse the motion, moving leg down past the SP and into a lunge, with chest up, hand reaching toward the sky (Fig. 4-80). After several repetitions, perform in like manner with left arm and leg, right side toward the wall. Kick high with knee straight, foot extended.

Take Turns. Repeat several sequences of four basic movements with four **Sway Forward and Back** movements.

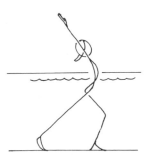

FIGURE 4-80

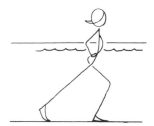

FIGURE 4-81

TRIGGERFISH

Firms stomach and buttocks. Variations add waist exercise.

GET SET: Stand with the left side toward the wall, left hand on the ledge, right hand on your hip. With legs in a lunge position (weight on left leg, knee bent; ball of right foot on floor in back, knee straight), lift your chest slightly and pull in your stomach (Fig. 4-81).

GO: Lift your right knee high to the front (Fig. 4-82), then press your leg back to the start. Perform briskly, pushing leg forcefully

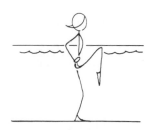

FIGURE 4-82

through the water. Keep your stomach pulled in. After several repetitions, reverse position and perform with the left leg.

VARIATIONS:

Touch Across—Point Back. This time, after lifting your right knee high to the front, swing your foot across in front, touching toes to the wall at the left (Fig. 4-83). Reverse the motion, swinging leg back to the SP. Perform briskly, pushing your leg forcefully through the water. In the beginning, touch your toes low on the wall; later, at surface level.

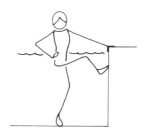

FIGURE 4-83

Take Turns. Perform several sequences combining eight basic movements done at a fast speed, with four of the previous variation done at a moderate speed. Or, using a moderate speed, alternate between the basic movement and the previous variation.

Body Slant. Make any of the **Triggerfish** movements more vigorous by doing them with your body on a slant. Stand with side toward the wall, several feet away. Lean toward the wall and hold the ledge with the inside hand, elbow straight. Put the other hand on your hip (Fig. 4-84).

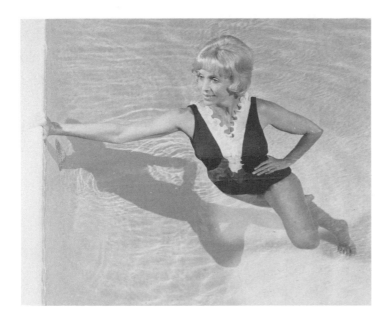

FIGURE 4-84

Trunk Shape-Ups While Suspended from the Pool Rim

Here is a group of Shape-Ups to do while suspended from the pool rim or ladder bars.[8] In this way, you can swing both legs simultaneously to firm muscles of the midsection, hips, and thighs and increase suppleness in your entire body. In addition, holding onto the rim or ladder strengthens hands, arms, and upper body (although you can expect some initial soreness in the arms as a result of holding these supports).

The first group of Suspended Shape-Ups is done facing the wall, the second group suspended with your back toward the wall. If you have a tendency to lordosis, the movements in this group are especially beneficial because they keep the lumbar area stretched while exercising the abdominal muscles in a shortened position. If they are available, ladder bars can be substituted for the rim for many movements in this section if their steps are recessed and the water is deep enough for your toes to clear the floor. Just hold them with elbows bent as shown in Fig. 4-III or grip them higher with elbows fully extended. When facing the wall, grip the bars with hands just above the water level.

If your pool lacks either a rim or ladder, or if supporting yourself at the wall is too stressful to your arms or shoulders, try doing **Feather Duster** movements from the "Stretchaway" chapter while supported by swim wings or kickboards. In addition, some of the movements in this section can be done using these floating supports, particularly **Dragonfly, Scud, Sandbug, Jollytail,** and **Pipefish.**

KNIFEFISH

Firms and strengthens all trunk muscles; stretches the trunk laterally

GET SET: Hold the pool rim or ladder bars and suspend yourself in **chin-deep water.** Hold the rim with hands slightly more than shoulder-width apart, fingers curled over the rim, base of hands braced against the wall. If you use the ladder, you can perform with your front or back toward the wall. Dangle your body straight down—buttocks tight, stomach in, feet extended and pressed together.

---

[8] Many of these Aquacises also can be done suspended from the end of a diving board. In fact, the **Barracuda** was developed especially for people who have their own pool and board.

GO: Swing your legs in a fishtail motion starting up to the right (Fig. 4-85), then down past the start and up to the left. For leverage, use a push-pull hand pressure; to bring legs to the right, press down with your right hand and push against the rim with your left hand. Reverse the pressure to move legs to the left. Repeat 10 to 15 times to each side.

REMEMBER: (1) Streamline your body by stretching. (2) Keep stomach pulled in, buttocks tight, and legs together. (3) Swing legs as high as possible. For maximum height, inhale and lean away from legs as they move up; exhale as they move down. (4) Avoid turning your hips—keep your front facing the wall.

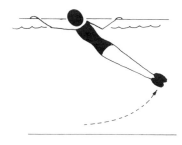

FIGURE 4-85

VARIATIONS:

Surface Fishtail. Perform the basic movement by swinging your legs horizontally, body at the surface. First, bring yourself into position by pressing elbows against the wall, then raise your legs to the surface in back—legs together, buttocks tight. When in position, straighten elbows and stretch out. Now you're ready to swing your legs from side to side by using arms in the push-pull style of the basic movement. *Caution—* those who are "weak of back" should skip this and the next variation.

Body Slant. Perform **Knifefish** in shallow water with your body cantilevered at an angle from the wall. On the downward motion, toes just clear the floor. If you need more leverage, brace your elbows against the wall (Fig. 4-86).

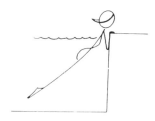

FIGURE 4-86

JOLLYTAIL

Firms and trims the abdomen. The first two variations add waist exercise.

GET SET: Face the pool wall in **shoulder-deep water** and hold the pool rim with hands slightly more than shoulder-width apart. Curl your fingers over the rim and brace the base of your hands against the wall. Suspend your body straight down— legs together, feet extended, toes touching the pool floor. Pull in your stomach and tighten your buttocks. To make this Aquacise more vigorous, suspend yourself in deeper water where your toes cannot reach the floor.

GO: Pump your knees vigorously up and down. (That is, lift them up to your chest, pulling in your stomach even more, Fig.

4-87, then push your legs down to the start.) Avoid jumping up—lift your knees instead.

VARIATIONS:

Knees Side. Continue the knee-pumping action, but this time lift them to the side. In a smooth, continuous motion, turn hips to face right, then lift knees toward the outside of the right shoulder (Fig. 4-88). Press legs down to the start, then repeat to the left. For more leverage, brace your left elbow against the wall as knees move up to the right; brace right elbow as knees move left.

Knees Around. Swing your knees in a circular motion. Start by 'ifting them toward your right shoulder; swing them under your right arm and across in front to the left, then down to the start (Fig. 4-89). After several repetitions, circle in the opposite direction. Pull in your stomach and lift knees high to the side and across in front as well.

Tummy Tuck. Hold the pool rim as instructed and perform the basic movement in **chest-deep water.** However, begin and end each "knees up" motion standing on tiptoe with feet *far* apart side to side (Fig. 4-90). Keep elbows straight, upper body still. Tuck up knees high in front, bringing legs together briefly before pushing them down and apart to the SP. Perform briskly.

PIPEFISH

Firms abdomen, hips, thighs, and buttocks. The last three variations add waist exercise.

GET SET: In **water at least chin deep,** face the wall and hold onto the pool rim with hands shoulder-width apart. For leverage, curl your fingers over the rim with thumbs and the base of the hands braced against the wall. Dangle your body straight down, legs together, stomach pulled in.

GO: Separate your legs, swinging them up to a high V-split (try to bring toes to the surface, Fig. 4-91) then press legs down to the start. At the height of the motion, bring toes close to the wall.

REMEMBER: (1) Push legs forcefully through the water, pulling in stomach even more as legs move up; tightening buttocks as legs move down. (2) Lift legs high, separating them as far as

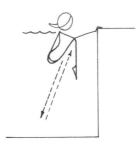

FIGURE 4-87

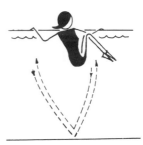

FIGURE 4-88

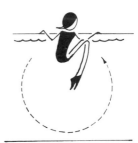

FIGURE 4-89

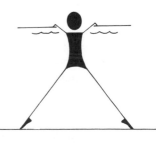

FIGURE 4-90

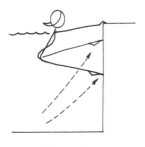

FIGURE 4-91

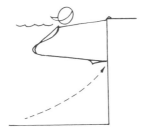

FIGURE 4-92

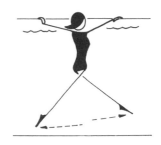

FIGURE 4-93

possible. (2) Keep legs stretched and feet extended. (3) Inhale as legs move up; exhale as they move down.

VARIATIONS:

Pike Up. This time, keep legs together and lift them forward at right angles to your body (Fig. 4-92). Then press legs down to the start. As legs move up, pull in your stomach even more and press hips back so that your toes clear the wall.

Take Turns. Alternate between the **Basic Pipefish** movement and the first variation.

"Pike-tail." Alternate between the first variation and the **Basic** or **Knees Side Jollytail** movements (p. 46).

"Pipe-tail." Alternate between **Basic Pipefish** and **Jollytail** movements.

Split Up—Turn. Perform the basic movement. However, instead of stopping the motion as legs come together, turn your hips to face right as you swing the left leg forward, right leg back. This puts your legs in a wide scissors split (Fig. 4-93). Next, turn to face the wall, bringing feet together. Repeat the sequence, this time turning left and swinging the right leg forward, left leg back. Stretch and tense legs and swing them far apart in both scissors and V-split positions.

SEA SQUIRT

Increases strength and flexibility of the anterior-posterior trunk and strengthens hands and arms

GET SET: In **shoulder-deep water,** face the wall and hold onto the pool rim with hands shoulder-width apart, elbows straight. Brace toes low on the wall, feet together (Fig. 4-94).

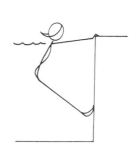

FIGURE 4-94

GO: In a smooth, forceful motion, bend elbows and pull your chest toward the wall as you swing your legs to the back (Fig. 4-95); then straighten elbows and push yourself backward as you swing legs forward to the start.

REMEMBER: (1) As you lift legs forward, pull in your stomach even more. Concentrate on making your abdominal muscles do the work. (2) As flexibility increases, strive to place feet higher on the wall as in Fig. 4-96. (3) Keep legs stretched, feet together. (4) Avoid bumping your chin when pulling forward.

VARIATION:

Arc Your Legs. Perform the basic movement, but instead of keeping legs together, separate them out to the side in a wide arc, bringing them together at the end of each forward and backward movement.

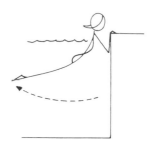

FIGURE 4-95

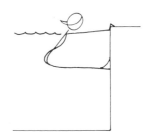

FIGURE 4-96

VENUS'S GIRDLE

Firms all muscles of the trunk, especially those of the abdominal girdle. Also increases trunk flexibility for a more supple body.

GET SET: Hold onto the pool rim or ladder bars and suspend yourself in **shoulder-deep water,** hands slightly more than shoulder-width apart. For leverage, curl your fingers over the rim and brace the base of your hands against the wall. Brace your toes low on the wall, feet together (Fig. 4-97). If using the ladder, brace toes on a lower rung.

GO: Swing your legs in a circle, ending with feet in the SP. To start each circle, lightly jump up pushing feet away from the wall; swing legs around to the back, over to the other side and forward to the SP. Periodically circle in the opposite direction.

REMEMBER: (1) Keep legs together, knees straight. (2) Pull in your stomach hard as you lift legs forward. Feel your abdominal muscles lifting your legs. (3) As strength and flexibility increase, enlarge the circle by bringing feet higher on the wall as in Fig. 4-96. (4) Avoid holding your breath.

VARIATION:

Part Company. This time, swing your legs in separate circles. Begin with arms in the **Get Set** position with body vertical,

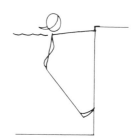

FIGURE 4-97

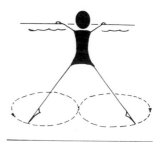

FIGURE 4-98

floating free. First, swing legs forward then separate them to the side; swing legs around to the back and together to the SP (Fig. 4-98). As legs move forward, pull your stomach in even more and press hips back so that feet clear the wall (Fig. 4-99).

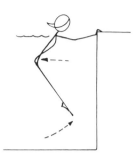

FIGURE 4-99

RIBBONFISH

Strengthens hands, arms, and all muscles of the trunk

GET SET: Face the wall and hold the pool rim securely with your hands slightly more than shoulder-width apart. Start with knees tucked under your right elbow, feet together and braced on the wall to the right (Fig. 4-100).

GO: Push your feet away from the wall, around to the back and across to the left, ending in a tucked position to the left (Fig. 4-101). Reverse the motion and swing around to the SP. In the beginning, you can keep your knees bent. Later, straighten them as you push off, then momentarily extend your body as your legs pass directly behind (Fig. 4-102). In either case, use your arms to help push away from the wall and pull toward it again at the other side. Start with 6 to each side and gradually increase to 12.

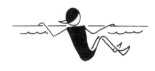

FIGURE 4-100

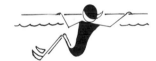

FIGURE 4-101

BULLFROG

Strengthens hands, arms, and all muscles of the trunk, especially the abdomen

GET SET: Face the wall and hold firmly onto the pool rim. With feet together, tuck your knees up and brace your toes on the wall in front (Fig. 4-103). Pull in your stomach.

GO: Release your hands, then immediately reach as far as possible to one side and grasp the pool rim. Next, vigorously push your feet away from the wall and around to the back; then tuck up your knees and bring feet forward to the wall. For easy coordination, repeat to yourself, "Reach, push, pull." (*Reach* hands to the side, *push* feet away, *pull* yourself into the tucked position.) Progress several yards in one direction, then reverse the motion and "jump" back to the start. Keep legs together and swing them high to the back; however, if you have a back problem, swing them low. Be sure to tuck knees energetically, keeping stomach pulled in.

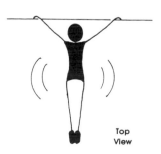

Top
View

FIGURE 4-102

DRAGONFLY

Firms abdomen, hips, and inner and outer thighs

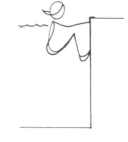

FIGURE 4-103

GET SET: Grasp the pool rim as shown in Fig. 4-104 with elbows straight and legs piked to bring toes close to the surface (feet should be higher than hips). For extra support, you can brace the back of your head or neck against the rim. Stretch and tense your legs, extend your feet, pull in your stomach. However, if this position is too stressful to your shoulders, you may (1) hold onto the ladder bars (Fig. 4-111) or (2) grip the pool rim with elbows bent, hands close to your ears (Fig. 4-105).

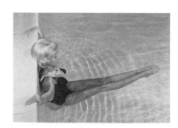

FIGURE 4-104

GO: Separate your legs to the side in a wide V-split, then press legs together, crossing them at the ankles (alternate right over left, then left over right, etc.). Repeat briskly a minimum of 15 times to a maximum of 40.

VARIATION:

Double Cross. Repeat several sequences of four slow **Dragon-flies** moving legs through a full range of motion, alternating with eight short, fast ones.

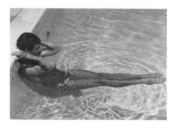

FIGURE 4-105

SCUD

Exercises waist, stomach, buttocks, and front/back of thighs.

GET SET: Start from any of the suspended positions suggested for **Dragonfly.** Lift legs forward to bring toes within 12 inches of the surface. With shoulders level, twist at the waist and roll to your left hip. Pull in your stomach, and stretch your legs with feet extended.

GO: Swing legs forward and back in a rapid scissors motion (Fig. 4-106). Swing them parallel to the surface and as far as possible to the front and back. Perform a minimum of 15 repetitions on each side to a maximum of 40.

VARIATION:

"Scud-fly." Combine **Scud** with **Dragonfly** as follows: Begin with legs together in **Dragonfly** SP, then open legs to a wide V-split. Next, roll onto your left hip and swing the right leg across to the left (Fig. 4-106). Roll onto your back, opening legs again to

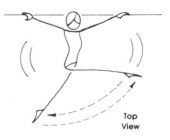

Top View

FIGURE 4-106

V-split. Roll onto the right hip and swing your left leg across. Move smoothly from one position into the next, swinging legs forcefully through their maximum range of motion.

SAND BUG

Exercises waist, abdomen, buttocks, and front/back of thighs

GET SET: Start from any of the suspended positions suggested for **Dragonfly.** Keeping shoulders level, roll onto the left hip with the side of your legs parallel to the surface. Pull in your stomach, stretch your legs, and extend your feet.

GO: Use your legs alternately in a brisk pedaling motion as though riding a bicycle (Fig. 4-107). Lift one knee at a time toward your chest; reach your foot far forward as you straighten the knee, then press your leg back against the water to the start. Exaggerate the movements keeping the side of legs parallel with the surface. Perform a minimum of 15 repetitions on each side to a maximum of 40.

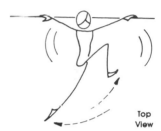

Top View

FIGURE 4-107

VARIATIONS:

Heels First. Perform **Sand Bug** with your feet flexed and push hard with your heels on the forward-back phase.

Heels 'n Toes. Pedal two times slowly with feet extended and four times quickly with your feet flexed. Repeat the sequence several times on each side. Roll quickly when changing from one side to the other without breaking the rhythm.

BARNACLE

Firms muscles of arms, abdomen, hips, buttocks, and thighs

GET SET: In **water at least shoulder deep,** suspend yourself as shown in Fig. 4-108, with elbows on the ledge, back flat against the wall. Pike legs forward, feet together, toes at the surface. At first, this arm position may be difficult to sustain. Therefore, perform the movement only a few times, change to a different Aquacise, then return to the suspended position and try again. It's also helpful to rest your elbows on a towel folded lengthwise.

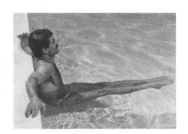

FIGURE 4-108

GO: Perform each of the following movements with your buttocks touching the wall. In addition, tighten buttocks as legs move down, then pull in stomach even more to bring lower back to the wall as legs move up. Stretch legs and swing them forcefully with feet extended.

Circle Side by Side. With legs together, swing them in large circles. For maximum circumference, (1) move them far to each side, (2) swing them up or down close to the wall, and (3) lift toes to the surface at the top of each loop.

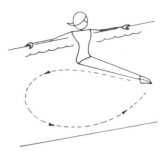

FIGURE 4-109

Circle One at a Time. Circle one leg at a time while stretching the other leg forward, toes at the surface. First, swing leg outward, then down close to the wall, touching heel to the wall before lifting leg foward to the start (Fig. 4-109). Circle repeatedly before changing legs or alternate legs after each circle. Periodically reverse direction of the circles.

Divide in Two. Swing your legs in separate circles. First, open legs to a wide V-split, then swing them down close to the wall bringing feet together, heels to the wall. Lift legs forward to the SP, (Fig. 4-110). Be sure to separate legs as far as possible in V-split, then tighten buttocks as legs move down. Periodically reverse direction of the circles. Also try this one at the ladder from the tight pike position shown in Fig. 4-111.

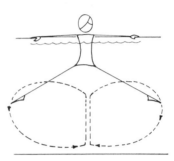

FIGURE 4-110

Half Circles. Perform **Divide in Two** until legs are vertical, heels touching the wall. Then reverse the motion, swinging legs apart and up to the SP.

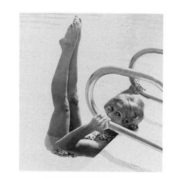

Scissors Up. This time, start with your left leg forward, toes at the surface, the right leg straight down, heel touching the wall. Now, exchange the position of your legs swinging them up and down vigorously in scissors fashion (Fig. 4-112). Keep your lower back against the wall.

FIGURE 4-111

Swirl Up. Begin in the **Scissors Up** SP. Moving legs simultaneously, exchange their position by swinging each leg outward and around in an arc (Fig. 4-113); then reverse the action to the SP. Move legs through the greatest possible range by constantly stretching them apart. Lift toes to the surface at the top of each arc and bring heel to the wall at the bottom. Keep lower back against the wall. Also try **Swirl Up** with feet flexed.

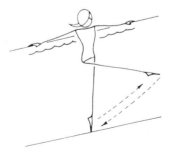

FIGURE 4-112

ANGLERFISH

Vigorous and challenging Aquacises to strengthen the abdomen and waist

GET SET: Grasp the pool rim with elbows straight as shown in Fig. 4-104. For extra support, you can brace the back of your head or neck against the rim. Lift your legs forward to an angle of 90°, toes close to the surface, feet together (hips float free without touching the wall). Better still, pike tighter to elevate your toes above the surface. Or, you can use an alternative SP shown in Fig. 4-108, with elbows on the ledge, hips against the wall.

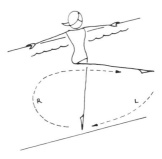

FIGURE 4-113

GO: To do each of these movements, pull in your stomach firmly, stretch legs with feet extended. Since the last two movements, and those done from a tight pike position at the ladder, are more strenuous, save them until your abdominal muscles have been conditioned by other Aquacises in this section.

Swing One by One. Swing your right leg out to the side while keeping the left leg in the SP. Swing leg forward to the start and repeat with the left leg. Try to swing leg out to the wall each time. You also can do this Aquacise holding the ladder. To make it even more difficult, start from the tight pike position in Fig. 4-111 and lower your legs to the surface at the side.

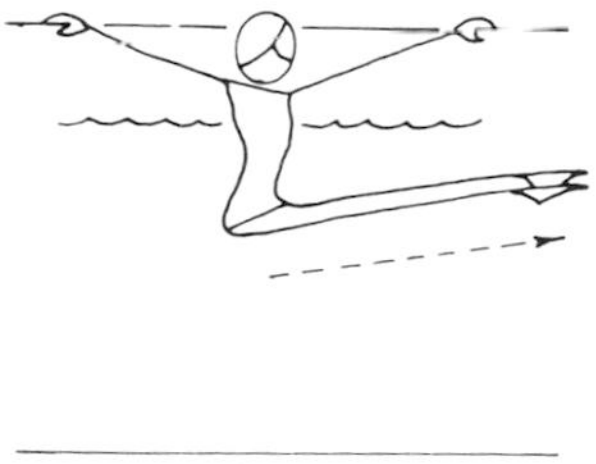

Swing Side by Side. With legs together, swing them from side to side (Fig. 4-114). Also try this version at the ladder. Better yet, start from the tight pike position in Fig. 4-111 and lower your legs to the surface at the side. Wow!

FIGURE 4-114

Swing Wide. Separate your legs into a wide V-split. Hold the split and swing legs from side to side. Try to touch the wall at each side with the furthermost foot.

Swing Twice. With legs in a wide V-split, swing them over to the right. Next, keeping right leg in place, swing the left leg across to meet it; swing left leg out to V-split and repeat the action to the left.

BARRACUDA

Strengthens and firms muscles of the trunk, hands, and arms;
stretches you from head to toe

GET SET: Swimmers, suspend yourself from the end of the diving board, hands gripping the sides of the board. Dangle your legs straight down, legs together, feet extended. Tighten buttocks and pull in your stomach.

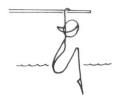

FIGURE 4-115

GO: Use the following Aquacises separately or combine them into a sequence by repeating each several times before moving onto the next.

Tuck and Arch. Tip your head forward and lift knees toward your chest until legs are in a tight tuck (Fig. 4-115). Next, extend legs down and back as you tip head back and arch your back (stretch legs, tighten buttocks, and lift chest, Fig. 4-116). Move smoothly from one position to the next, keeping stomach pulled in.

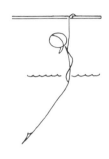

FIGURE 4-116

Pike and Arch. Lift your legs forward, knees straight, bringing toes to the surface. At the same time press hips back (Fig. 4-117). Next, press hips forward as you swing legs down and back into an arched position (Fig. 4-116). Swing smoothly back and forth, keeping stomach pulled in and legs together. Later, when abdominal muscles are stronger, pike sharply and lift toes to the level of the board (Fig. 4-118) instead of just bringing your toes to the surface of the water.

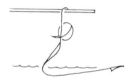

Arc Your Legs. Perform **Pike and Arch** but, instead of keeping legs together, swing them apart to the side. Then, bring them together at the end of each forward and backward movement.

FIGURE 4-117

Twist—Tuck. With hips turned to face right, pump your knees up and down several times, then repeat with hips turned to the left.

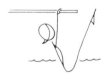

Twist—Tuck—Swing. Turn your hips to the right. Now, lift knees toward your right shoulder, then swing them across in front toward your left shoulder; extend legs down to the SP. Repeat to the left side. Alternate sides. Lift knees high as you swing them across, keeping stomach pulled in.

Circle on Three Levels.

Low. Keeping body vertical, circle legs as in Fig. 4-98.

FIGURE 4-118

Medium. Start with legs forward, toes at the surface. Now, swing them apart to a wide V-split; press them down and together, then lift them forward to the start. After several repetitions, circle in the opposite direction.

High (difficult). Begin and end each circle in the tight pike position in Fig. 4-118. This is extremely vigorous and should only be used if your abdominal muscles have been conditioned by other Aquacises.

Lower Limb Shape-Ups

Overeating and underexercising are the primary causes of flabby hips, thighs, and buttocks, as well as excessive fat deposits in these areas. Other contributing factors are the cumulative effects of gravitational force and the hormonal changes that occur as one grows older. (Alas, after age 25, active muscle tissue gradually decreases and fat increases.) However, with Lower Limb Shape-Ups, muscles in these areas can be conditioned and flabby tissue made more firm and compact. Toward this goal, I have developed a galaxy of Aquacises that are among my students' favorites and will appeal to you too, especially since they are done in the cool, comfortable water.

During this group of "cool kicks," you will swing your legs in a variety of ways against the water's resistance. Each Aquacise involves muscular action in both legs and your trunk as well. The muscles most involved in moving your working leg contract concentrically while the muscles of your supporting leg and trunk contract to stabilize you against the water's opposing force. Further, the more speed, force, and range of motion you apply with your working leg, the greater the water's counterforce, and the harder the muscles of both legs must work.

In addition to helping you acquire trim, shapely hips and thighs, Lower Limb Shape-Ups will:

1. Aid your posture by strengthening some of those important antigravity muscles that help to hold you erect on land (i.e., muscles of the anterior thighs, buttocks, abdomen and back).
2. Increase flexibility of hip joints, hamstrings (posterior thighs), ankles, and feet.

As an added bonus, firm leg muscles also support the veins and aid the return of venous blood back to the heart

Lower Limb Shape-Ups

against the force of gravity. Our legs have been called the body's auxiliary heart because their muscular contractions during exercise further stimulate blood flow upward. So, pick your favorite Lower Limb Aquacises and get busy. Our legs are important—they keep us upright *and* mobile!

Unless advised otherwise, start with 10 repetitions of each of your chosen Lower Limb Shape-Ups and work up to 30. Be sure to perform Lower Limb Shape-Ups in a like manner with the opposite leg.

DAPHNIA

Firms abdomen, buttocks, lower back, front and back of thighs. Also stretches the back and back of legs.

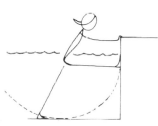

FIGURE 4-119

GET SET: In chest-deep water, stand facing the wall about 2½ feet out. Lean forward on a slant and hold the ledge with elbows straight. Extend your right leg up to the back and pull in your stomach.

GO: Swing your leg down and up to the front, flexing your foot (Fig. 4-119), then swing leg down and back to the start. Keep knees straight with heel of supporting foot on the floor. Foot of working leg may be flexed throughout or extended during the backward motion. Strive to bring toes to the surface in front, heel to the surface in back, keeping leg stretched/tensed.

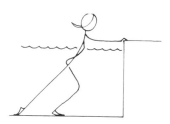

FIGURE 4-120

VARIATIONS:

Touch Down. Stand in the **Get Set** position on the ball of your left foot. Swing your right leg forward and back, then bend left knee as you press the right leg down, touching toes to the floor in back (Fig. 4-120). Straighten left knee as you kick right leg up to the back, then repeat the entire movement several times. Keep stomach pulled in, elbows straight. Touch toes to the floor as far back as possible.

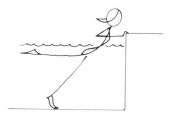

FIGURE 4-121

Push—Pull. Stand on the ball of your left foot to perform the basic movement and, as right leg moves back, bend elbows to bring chest toward the wall (Fig. 4-121); straighten them as leg moves forward (Fig. 4-119).

HATCHETFISH

Firms and trims hips, buttocks, and inner and outer thighs

GET SET: Face the pool wall and stand arms' length away, hands on the ledge in front. Or, stand with your left side toward the wall and hold the ledge with your left hand. Turn your left foot out about 45°. Lift your right leg out to the side, knee cap facing up (rotate leg outward at the hip joint), foot flexed (Fig. 4-122).

GO: Using crisp movements, press your right leg down and across in front of the left, brushing heel close to the floor (Fig. 4-123). Lift leg sideward and repeat, this time crossing leg in back.

REMEMBER: (1) Stretch your working leg and maintain its outward rotation to keep knee and foot in a fixed position. (2) Keep heel of supporting foot on the floor.

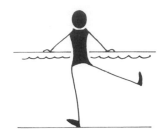

FIGURE 4-122

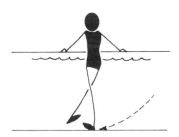

FIGURE 4-123

WATER WITCH

Leg movement firms muscles of lower body as well as front and back of thighs. Arm movement tones arms and upper body.

GET SET: Stand in **waist-to-chest-deep water** with your right side toward the wall, right hand holding the ledge (or rest your elbow on the ledge as in Fig. 4-124). Hold your left arm forward, hand just under the surface, and lift your left leg to the back. Lean forward to bring your leg high and stretch from fingertips to toes (Fig. 4-125).

GO: Swing your arm down and back as you swing your leg down and forward (Fig. 4-126) then reverse the motion back to the SP. Do **Water Witch** with foot either flexed or extended. Better yet, do eight movements with foot in each position and repeat this sequence two or more times.

REMEMBER: (1) Stretch and tense working leg and try to kick up to the surface. (2) Palm may face backward the entire time or turned to face forward during the forward motion. In either case, dig arm forcefully into the water. (3) If coordination is difficult, omit the arm motion at first.

VARIATIONS:

Kick Diagonal. Stand erect, left side toward the wall, arms' length away. Hold the ledge with the left hand, right hand on

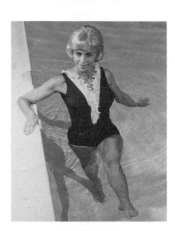

FIGURE 4-124

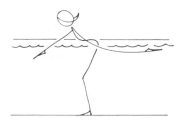

FIGURE 4-125

hip. Now, omitting the arm swing, perform the basic kick moving your right leg *diagonally* forward toward the wall, then backward along the same path. Be sure to keep hips facing front and swing leg with knee cap always turned out (rotate leg outward at the hip joint).

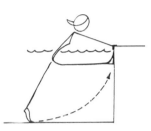

FIGURE 4-126

DIPPER

A three-way kick to exercise all muscles of the lower trunk and thighs and put you in (s)hip shape

GET SET: Face the wall and stand arms' length away, hands on the ledge in front. Stand tall with feet together.

GO: Use the following movements separately or in sequence by repeating each several times before moving to the next.

Kick Front. Kick your right leg forward with your foot flexed. Press your leg down and repeat with the left leg. At the height of the kick, touch the sole of your foot to the wall (Fig. 4-127). If you have a low-back problem, lift your leg with the knee bent and touch only your toes to the wall. Otherwise try to keep both knees straight.

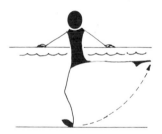

FIGURE 4-127

Kick Side Kick your right leg up to the side with your foot either flexed or extended (Fig. 4-128), then press it down to the start and repeat with the left leg. For a bouncy effect, bend your supporting knee as working leg moves up; straighten it as leg moves down.

Kick Back. Kick your right leg back, press it down to the start, and repeat with the left leg. As you kick back, bend your elbows and lean forward slightly to bring your leg high (Fig. 4-129). As you press your leg down, stand upright again. Kick back with foot either flexed or extended.

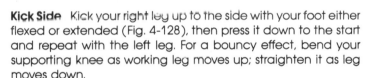

FIGURE 4-128

GRUNT

Exercises all muscles of lower trunk and thighs

GET SET: Stand in **chest-deep water** facing the wall about three feet out. Lean forward on a slant and hold the ledge with elbows straight.

GO: In a smooth, continuous motion, lift your left leg to the back; then swing it around to the left side and forward toward

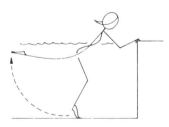

FIGURE 4-129

the wall (Fig. 4-130). Next, swing your leg back along the same path, then press it down to the start. Perform with foot extended or, for variation, with foot flexed.

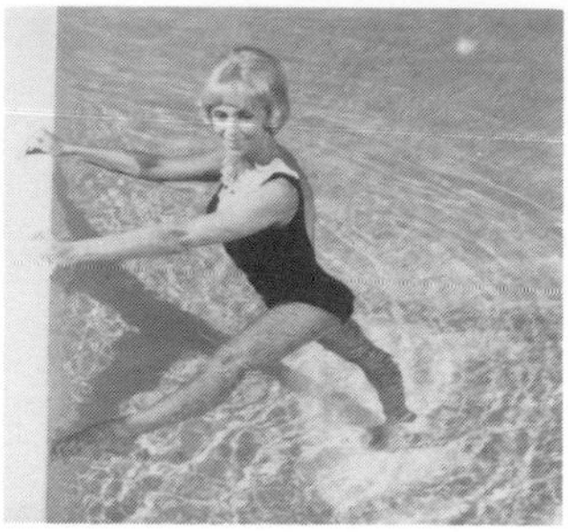

REMEMBER: (1) Swing leg forward just under and parallel to the surface of the water with knee straight. (2) Coax leg higher in back just before pressing it down to the SP. (3) Heel of supporting foot may remain on the floor for an extra stretch in back of leg.

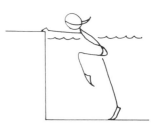

VARIATIONS:

FIGURE 4-130

Ditto. Keeping leg elevated, swing it forward and back several times before pressing it down to the start.

Add a Knee Lift. Between each basic movement, bend knee of working leg up to chest (Fig. 4-131) then return leg to the start. Move smoothly through this sequence without pausing.

Hop 'n Change. Do the **Grunt** with alternate legs, but omit bringing leg down to the start each time. Instead, substitute a hop (when leg is back) to change from one to the other.

Push—Pull. Bend elbows to bring chest toward the wall as leg moves back; straighten them as leg moves forward.

FIGURE 4-131

Reverse Gear. This time, start by lifting leg forward (flex your foot to clear the wall), swing leg around to the side and back, then swing it forward and down to the start. Flex foot throughout or extend it during the sideward motion.

Once Forward—Once Back. Alternate basic with **Reverse Gear** movements.

"COUNTING" CORMORANT

Strengthens and firms hips, buttocks, abdomen, and all areas of the thighs

GET SET: Stand tall with your back close to the wall in **waist-to-chest-deep water.** Hold the ledge with arms sideward and pull in your stomach.

GO: Raise your right leg forward and draw large numbers from one to ten with your toes, then trace all ten numbers again by counting back. Swing your leg from the hip through a large range of motion, with your knee straight, foot extended.

VARIATIONS:

Other Choices. In addition to numbers only, try writing the alphabet or your name and address.

Show Off. Repeat several sequences of **"Counting" Cormorant** alternating with **"Smart Smelt"** (p. 34.) Move into **"Smart" Smelt** SP by stepping forward on one foot to bring feet apart front to back.

FANFISH

Firms and trims all trunk and thigh muscles

GET SET: Face the pool wall and suspend yourself in **water at least shoulder deep.** Hold onto the pool rim and brace your right foot midway up the wall, knee bent. Or, brace your right foreleg against the wall as in Fig. 4-132. Elevate your left leg high to the side, foot extended, toes touching the wall. (Try to lift toes to the surface.)

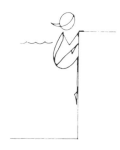

FIGURE 4-132

GO: Swing your left leg in a wide arc, first out to the side, then across and down in back touching foot to the wall at the right (Fig. 4-133). Reverse the motion and return leg to the start. Keep knee of working leg straight, stomach pulled in. Avoid holding your breath.

JEWELFISH

Firms and trims abdomen, hips, buttocks, and thighs

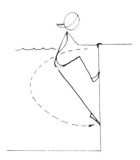

GET SET: Stand in **waist-to-chest-deep water** with your back close to the wall, feet together, stomach pulled in. Hold arms sideward and rest your hands on the ledge.

FIGURE 4-133

GO: Kick your right leg diagonally forward to the left, press it down to the start, then kick diagonally foward to the right and return (Fig. 4-134). For a bouncy effect, bend supporting knee as leg moves up; straighten it as leg moves down. Repeat several times before changing to the left leg or alternate legs. Keep hips facing forward and kick high with knee straight, foot extended.

VARIATIONS:

Wallflower. Stand with your left side toward the wall. Hold the ledge with your left hand and put the right hand on your hip.

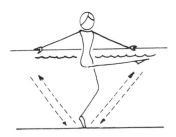

FIGURE 4-134

Perform **Jewelfish** with the right leg (Fig. 4-135) and, instead of returning to a feet-together position each time, press your leg down and back to a lunge (weight on left leg, knee bent; ball of right foot on the floor in back; knee straight, Fig. 4-136). Keep hips facing forward, stomach in, back erect.

Body Slant. Stand facing the wall 2½ feet out. Lean forward and hold the ledge with body and elbows straight. Now, perform **Jewelfish** with the right leg, keeping foot flexed. As you kick diagonally right, touch your toes to the wall at the right, then press leg down and back to a lunge position (Fig. 4-137). Next, kick diagonally left, touching toes to the wall at the left. Repeat several times before changing to the left leg or omit the lunge and bring feet together instead, then alternate legs. Keep working knee straight, stomach pulled in.

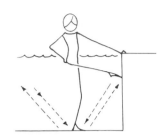

FIGURE 4-135

SWEEPER

Firms hips, buttocks, lower back, and all thigh muscles

GET SET: Stand in **waist-to-chest-deep water** either with left side toward the wall holding the ledge with left hand or, face the wall, hands on the ledge, arms' length away. Stand tall.

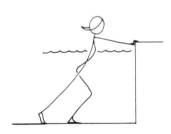

FIGURE 4-136

GO: These Aquacises may be used separately or combined into a sequence in which each is repeated several times before moving on to the next.

Floor Sweep. Start with the left knee bent, right leg diagonally across in front, toes touching the floor. Now, sweep your right leg outward and around to the other side by tracing a wide arc on the floor with your toes (Fig. 4-138); then reverse the motion around to the start.

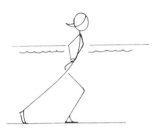

FIGURE 4-137

Half Mast. Swing your leg horizontally as in **Floor Sweep** but with your foot elevated to knee level (Fig. 4-139).

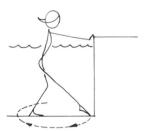

FIGURE 4-138

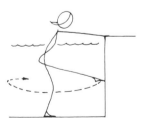

FIGURE 4-139

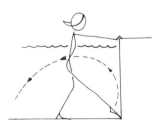

FIGURE 4-140

Sweep Up—Touch Down. Start as in **Floor Sweep,** but this time swing your leg in an arc up to the side, then down and across in back to a lunge position (weight on left leg, knee bent; ball of right foot on floor in back, knee straight). Reverse the motion and sweep your leg around to the start. Begin with small arcs; later, bring your foot up to the surface at the side, (Fig. 4-140). Remember to flex your foot on the forward phase to avoid bumping toes on the wall. And, each time your leg moves up, straighten your supporting knee and rise high onto the ball of your foot; bend your knee again as your leg moves down.

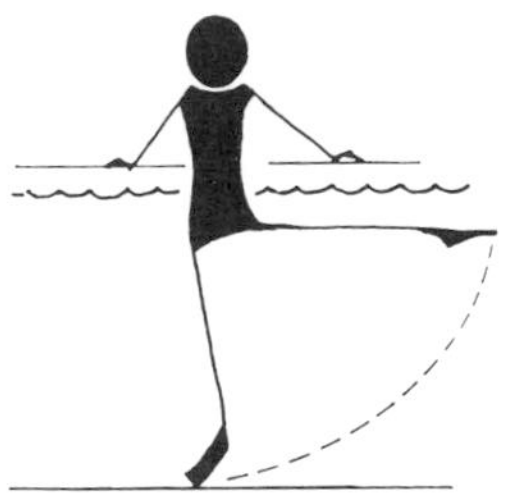

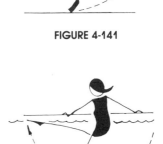

FIGURE 4-141

Remember: (1) Strive for the largest arcs possible by crossing your leg far over, both in front and in back. (2) Keep back straight while swinging leg from the hip. (3) Keep stomach in, working knee straight.

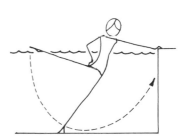

FIGURE 4-142

SWORDTAIL

Another vigorous leg movement to smooth and firm contours of hips, thighs, and abdomen and increase flexibility of hip joints

GET SET: Stand on the balls of your feet in **waist-to-chest-deep water** with your back or front facing the wall. Stand tall and hold the ledge with arms sideward.

GO: Kick your right leg sideward (Fig. 4-141) then swing it down, across in front, and up to the left (Fig. 4-142). Reverse the motion swinging leg down and up to the side, then down to the feet-together SP.

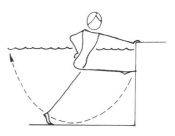

FIGURE 4-143

REMEMBER: (1) Move leg directly to each side. Kick out to the right with knee cap facing up (turn leg out at the hip), hips facing forward. Kick across turning hips left. (2) Kick high with foot extended to bring toes to the surface at each side.

VARIATIONS:

Body Slant. Stand in **chest-deep water** with your left side toward the wall about three feet out. Lean toward the wall on a slant and hold the ledge with your left hand, elbow straight. Put your right hand on your hip. Perform **Swordtail** with the right leg and try to lift your toes above the surface at the right (Fig. 4-143) then touch them high on the wall at the left (Fig. 4-144). Apply Reminder (1) given above for the basic movement.

FIGURE 4-144

HIP-POPOTAMUS

Provides Swordtail benefits and exercises calves and feet as well

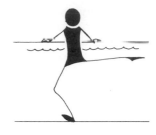

FIGURE 4-145

GET SET: In **waist-to-chest-deep water,** face the wall and hold onto the ledge arms' length away. Stand erect on your left foot, left knee bent. Raise your right leg high to the side, knee cap facing up, foot extended close to the surface (Fig. 4-145). Now you're ready to do this two-part sequence 12 to 20 times with each leg.

GO: (1) Swing your leg down, across in front, and up to the surface at the left as shown in Fig. 4-142; then reverse the motion swinging leg down and up to the side SP. (2) Leap up and over to the right, landing on your right foot (Figs. 4-146 and 4-147). Immediately leap over to the left, landing on your left foot. Now, with your right leg sideward in the SP, you're ready to repeat this sequence several times before changing to the other leg.

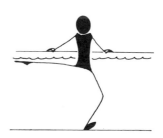

FIGURE 4-146

REMEMBER: (1) Apply the **Swordtail** reminders. (2) Leap far to each side, bending supporting knee as you land and lifting other leg high to the side. You can use your arms to help lift and support you.

VARIATIONS:

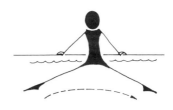

FIGURE 4-147

Stacatto. In **chest-deep water,** repeat several sequences of the following: do Part (1) of **Hip-Popotamus** four times, then pump right leg down and up eight times (that is, touch toes to the floor at the side, Fig. 4-148, and lift leg sideward again). *Remember:* (1) Keep working knee straight, supporting knee bent. (2) Touch toes down far to the side. (3) Try to kick up to the surface at the side. (4) Keep back erect and body still—confine all the action to the working leg.

Take Turns. Alternate between one **Hip-Popotamus** Part (2) and one down-up **Stacatto** motion. Repeat this sequence several times before changing to the other leg.

Side View. Perform the basic movement with left side facing the wall, left hand holding the ledge. Extend right arm sideward, hand just under the surface. As you leap to the right, release the ledge; as you leap left, grasp the ledge again. Keep back erect, stomach pulled in.

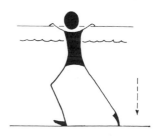

FIGURE 4-148

SNAPPER

Strengthens and firms calves and front/back of thighs, especially the area in front, just above the knee

GET SET: Stand in **waist-to-chest-deep water** with your back close to the wall, arms sideward, hands on the ledge. Bend your right knee and put the sole of your foot against the wall (Fig. 4-149). Stand tall and pull in your stomach.

GO: Swing your lower leg forward, staightening your knee (Fig. 4-150) then bend knee and push foot back to the wall. Kick up wIth foot either extended, flexed, or completely relaxed.

REMEMBER: (1) Straighten your knee sharply. (2) As you do, jab the surface with your toes, flicking the water upward.

VARIATIONS:

Snap Side. Face the wall arms' length away and hold onto the ledge. Stand on your left foot (turn it out 45°) and lift your right leg sideward, knee cap facing up. Now, bend and straighten your right knee, pushing your foot down behind the left knee. thon lifting it to the surface at the side. For a greater stretch to inner thighs, use the suggested SP, but let your weight fall to the right to bring legs apart to maximum stretch. Perform **Snap Side** from this position (Fig. 4-151). Keep stomach pulled in.

Snap Forward—Snap Side. Stand with your left side toward the wall. Using the right leg, perform **Snapper** alternately kicking forward (knee facing forward), then sideward (knee facing the side). Or, bend and straighten knee several times before changing direction. With each kick, lift toes to the surface, then swing foot down past left knee. Change direction of kick as foot moves up.

FIREFLY

Firms front and back of thighs, abdomen, buttocks, and calves

Firefly is similar to punting a football and combines the hip joint action of **Water Witch** with the knee action of **Snapper.**

GET SET: Stand in **waist-to-chest-deep water** with your left side toward the wall. Hold the ledge with your left hand and put your right hand on your hip.

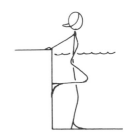

FIGURE 4-149

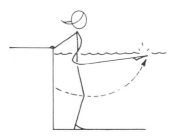

FIGURE 4-150

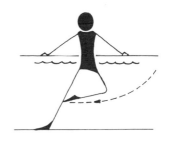

FIGURE 4-151

GO: Swing your right leg forward and back. As you do, bend your knee to bring your heel close to the surface at the height of the backward motion; straighten knee as you swing leg down and forward (Fig. 4-152).

REMEMBER: (1) **Firefly** is a sequential action which begins in the hip joint then moves to the knee with the foot following through on the final phase. (2) Move through a full range of motion at the hip joint and (3) forcefully bend and straighten your knee.

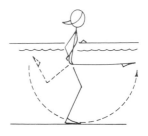

FIGURE 4-152

VARIATIONS:

Combination. Kick right leg forward, then bend knee and swing foot across in front of left knee. Straighten leg forward again, then swing leg back bending knee at height of swing. Coordinate the action by repeating to yourself, "Swing forward, across, forward, back."

Knee Diagonal. Perform **Firefly** kicking forward on a diagonal plane. Alternate kicking first to the right, then to the left. Repeat the sequence several times.

The next three Aquacises—**Discus, Whirligig,** and **Loon**—are comprised of leg-circling movements, any of which will firm all muscles of the lower trunk and thighs and increase flexibility in hip joints as well. For maximum benefits, do as many different ones as time and energy permit. Just remember to (1) move legs through the greatest possible circumference, (2) pull in your stomach, and (3) stretch/tense your working leg from thigh to extended foot.

DISCUS

GET SET: Stand in **waist-to-chest-deep water** using the starting positions given for the various Aquacises below.

GO: You can begin with any leg circles in this group and move to deeper water for the last two.

Round 'n Round. Stand with your back close to the wall, arms sideward, hands on the ledge. Starting with leg forward, circle leg four times each in small, medium, then large circles (Fig. 4-153) for a total of 12. Repeat in reverse direction. Perform briskly and do the sequence two or more times.

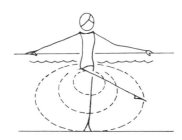

FIGURE 4-153

Circle Front. Stand tall with your back close to the wall, arms sideward, hands on the ledge. Now, swing one leg in large circles to the front (Fig. 4-154). Repeat several times, then change legs or alternate legs after each repetition. Periodically (1) circle in the opposite direction and (2) circle with your foot flexed.

Circle Back. Stand facing the wall about three feet out. Lean forward on a slant and hold the ledge with elbows straight. Lift your left leg to the back (Fig. 4-155). Now, swing your leg in large circles to the back, repeating several times with each leg or alternate legs after each repetition. Periodically circle in the opposite direction.

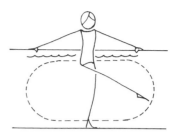

FIGURE 4-154

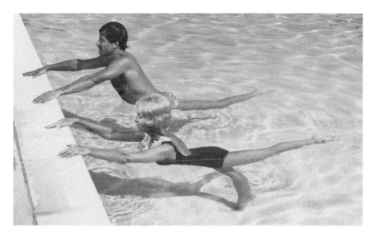

FIGURE 4-155

About Face. Repeat **Circle Front** eight times with the right leg. Then, on the downward phase of the last circle, turn left to face the wall and, without pausing, move leg right into **Circle Back** eight times. Repeat the sequence with left leg and turn right to face the wall. Work up until you can repeat the sequence three times.

Circle Side. Face the wall arms' length away and hold onto the ledge. Stand tall with the left foot turned out 45°. Raise the right leg sideward, knee cap facing up, extended foot at the surface. Tuck-in. Now you're ready to swing your leg in large circles to the side (brush toes lightly to the wall on the forward motion and to the floor on the down motion; then swing leg back before lifting it to the side SP, Fig. 4-156). Keep back erect,

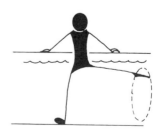

FIGURE 4-156

hips facing forward. After several repetitions, circle in the other direction. To vary, circle with foot flexed.

Circle Front—Toes Up. Stand facing the wall about three feet out. Lean forward on a slant and hold the ledge with elbows straight. Now, swing your leg in large circles to the front with foot flexed (follow the outline of a large, imaginary circle drawn on the wall (Fig. 4-157). After several repetitions, circle in the opposite direction.

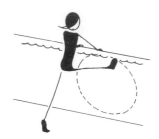

FIGURE 4-157

Circle—Touch. Stand facing the wall about three feet out. Lean forward on a slant and hold the ledge with elbows straight. Brace your right foot on the wall about halfway up. (As you gain flexibility, place your sole high on the wall with toes at the surface, knee straight.) Now, swing your leg in large circles, pausing in the SP at the end of each one to stretch your leg (Fig. 4-158). Keep heel of supporting foot on the floor and swing leg through the greatest possible range. (Swing down past supporting leg, up high to the back, or front, and around to the surface at the side.) After several repetitions, circle in the other direction.

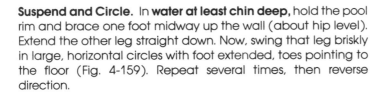

FIGURE 4-158

Suspend and Circle. In **water at least chin deep,** hold the pool rim and brace one foot midway up the wall (about hip level). Extend the other leg straight down. Now, swing that leg briskly in large, horizontal circles with foot extended, toes pointing to the floor (Fig. 4-159). Repeat several times, then reverse direction.

Extended Range. Suspend yourself as suggested above, but with working leg sideward, toes close to the surface. This time, swing your leg in giant ovals, bringing foot forward toward the wall, down across in back, then back and up to the side SP (Fig. 4-160).

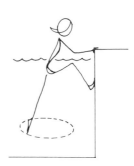

FIGURE 4-159

WHIRLIGIG

GET SET: Stand at the pool wall in **waist-to-chest-deep water** using the starting positions suggested below.

GO: Do either one or both of these horizontal figure-eight movements.

Circle Eight. Stand tall with your back close to the wall, arms sideward, hands resting on the ledge. Make the first loop by swinging your right leg across to the left, up to the surface, around to the front, then down past your left leg. Move right

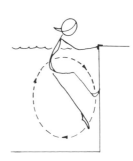

FIGURE 4-160

into the second loop by swinging leg out to the right side, up to the surface, around to the front, and down again (Fig. 4-161). Do some **Circle Eights** with your foot flexed. Even better, do four complete movements with foot extended, then four more with foot flexed. Repeat this sequence two or more times.

Circle Eight—Toes Up. Stand facing the wall about three feet out. Lean forward on a slant and hold the ledge with elbows straight. Lift your right leg sideward. To make the first loop, press leg down past the left leg and up to the front (flex foot to avoid bumping the wall), then out to the side SP. Make the second loop by pressing leg down, up to the back, and around to the side (Fig. 4-162). Perform as suggested or, instead of one circle in front and one in back, circle twice. When doing **Circle Eight—Toes Up,** remember: (1) Begin each loop with leg sideward, toes close to the surface. (2) The first action for each loop is to swing leg down past supporting leg.

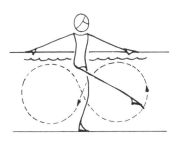

FIGURE 4-161

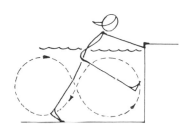

FIGURE 4-162

LOON

GET SET: Stand at the wall in **waist-to-chest-deep water** using the various starting positions suggested below.

GO: Swing your leg tracing giant loops with your toes.

Uplift Your Sole. Stand on the balls of your feet facing the wall about three feet out. Lean forward on a slant and hold the ledge with elbows straight. Brace your right foot about halfway up the wall. (Work to eventually place it high on the wall with toes at the surface, knee straight.) First, swing your leg in a large circle, pressing it down, up to the back, then around to the side and forward. Without pausing, swing leg down and up to the back (Fig. 4-163). Now you're in position to reverse the motion by kicking down and up to the front, to the side and back, then down and up to the forward SP.

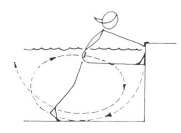

FIGURE 4-163

Remember: (1) Kick high to the front and back and sweep leg close to the surface at the side. (2) Flex your foot on the forward motion to avoid bumping the wall.

Swoop. Start with your back close to the wall, arms sideward, hands on the ledge. Lift your right leg out to the side. First, swing it down and across to the left, then in a large circle up to the surface in front, around to the side, then down and up to the left (Fig. 4-164). Reverse the motion, swinging leg down and up

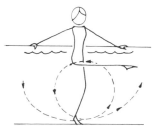

FIGURE 4-164

to the right, then circle across in front and around to the SP at the right.

Change Course. Stand on the balls of your feet facing the wall about three feet out. Lean forward on a slant and hold the ledge with elbows straight. Lift your right leg up to the back. Start by swinging your leg down and up to the front, then swing it out to the right and down across to the left (Fig. 4-165). Reverse the action by swinging down and up to the right, forward toward the wall, then straight down and back to the SP. Apply **Uplift Your Sole** reminders (the first Aquacise in this group).

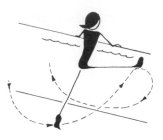

FIGURE 4-165

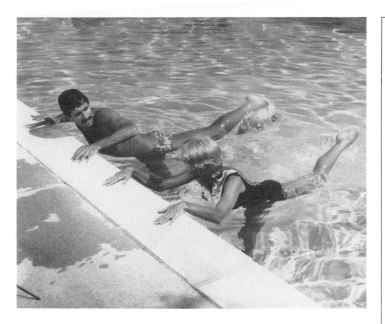

Here's a series of bright, lively movements that literally "take a load off your feet"—and you don't have to swim a stroke! They'll give you strong, supple, Happy Feet; pep up your cardiovascular system; firm your skeletal muscles, especially those of your feet, legs and trunk; and tone your midsection through deep breathing. On top of all this, they provide two additional bonuses. They burn calories faster because of the energy required to overcome the water's resistance and, as one student put it, "jumping and jogging in the water don't rattle your bones." In other words, the water virtually eliminates impact on the joints.

This chapter is divided into several groups: **Snail**—using numerous ways of walking in the shallow water; **Lily Trotter**—using jogging and running movements; **Dolphin**—using jumping movements; **Sand Hopper**—using hopping movements; and **Salmon**—using kicking movements while holding onto the side of the pool.

These Aquacises are an important part of your Water Workouts. Use them nonstop for at least two minutes at a time between other Aquacises, and for longer periods for increased circulatory/respiratory endurance as explained in "Why and How to Aquacise Aerobically." Here are some ways of combining them to help you move nonstop and to keep your sessions always fun:

1. Move across the pool using one style of locomotion, return using another.

Walk, Jog, Jump, Hop, and Kick Aquacises

SNAIL (p. 73)
  Step Long
  Step Lively
  Teeny Tiny Forward Steps
  Lift Knee and Push
  High Step
  High Step and Twist
  Step—Kick
  Poker Walk
  Kick and Lunge
  Clap Down
  Reach One Arm Forward
  Reach Both Arms Forward
  Reach Up and Over
  Kick Across—Lunge Side
  Step Across
  Extended Range
  Lift Knee Across
  Step Backward
  Kick Back and Step
  Teeny Tiny Backward Steps
  Slide Wide to the Side
  Lift—Press
  Slide 'n Arch
  Reach Side—Swing Across
  Circle 'n Slide
  Scamper Side

LILY TROTTER (p. 78)
  Jog Free
  Jog at the Wall
  Toes Up
  Pitter—Patter
  Run!
  Smooth Sailing
  Run Upstream

DOLPHIN (p. 82)
  Pop Up—Feet Together
  Open—Close
  Pop Overs
  Pop 'n Twist
  Pop Backward—Forward
  Pop Side to Side

  Pop Up—Feet Apart
  Close—Open
  Swing
  Squirt
  Flapdoodle
  Hot Foot
  Pop 'n Whirl
  Flying High
  Pop 'n Cross
  Jump 'n Lunge
  Scissor Legs
  Double Time
  Pop Forward
  Pop Backward
  Pop Sideward
  Spurt
  Kick Up—Pop Forward
  Bounce on the Wall
  Rise and Shine

SAND HOPPER (p. 87)
  Forward Hop
  Hold Your Foot 'n Hop
  Bun-ny Hop
  Hold Your Thigh 'n Hop
  Backward Hop
  Sideward Hop
  Sideward Hop—Pump Knee
  Make It Snappy
  Hop Kick to the Front
  Scuttle
  Hop Kick Your Hands
  Hop Kick 'n Tilt
  Hop Kick to the Back
  Hop Kick Your Backside
  Rock Forward and Back
  Rock Side to Side
  Hippety—Hop
  Leap for Joy!

SALMON (p. 92)
  Just for Kicks
  Lickety-Split
  V-Split and Cross

2. Combine two or three movements into a sequence by re-peating each one 10 times or so before moving onto the next. Repeat the sequence across several widths of the pool.

3. Intersperse movements, singly or in groups of two or three, between Shape Up, Paddle, or Beach Ball Aquacises, or between laps of swimming strokes or kicking with a kickboard.

4. Move across four widths of the pool as follows: for the first width, move forward by walking, jogging, etc; return moving sideways (as in **Scamper Side** (p. 78) or **Pop Sideward** (p. 85); for the third crossing, move backward by swimming on your back, hopping, or walking, etc.; return moving sideways with the other side leading. For longer trips, repeat this sequence two or more times.

5. Intersperse movements done in place (such as **Jog at the wall** (p. 79), **Squirt** (p. 83), or **Bun-ny Hop** (p. 88) with those that move you across the pool.

As you briskly move along, lift your chest, stretch your body and legs, and pull in your stomach. Slow down as necessary to avoid overexertion. These are the ways to get the most out of "Walk, Jog, Jump, Hop, and Kick" Aquacises.

SNAIL

GET SET: For these walking movements, start to one side of the pool in water between **waist and lower-chest level.** Avoid deeper water because buoyancy reduces your traction and makes it difficult to move forcefully.

GO: Walk back and forth across the pool using as many of these movements as time and energy permit. Be sure to swing your legs forcefully against the water's resistance and push your feet firmly against the floor for momentum; keep your back straight, shoulders relaxed, stomach pulled in; and avoid holding your breath.

Step Long. Lean forward slightly and walk with giant steps across the pool (see how few steps you need to get across). With each step, land on your heel, roll up to the ball of your foot, then firmly push off with your toes.

Use any of these arm positions: (a) hands on hips, (b) palms on the back of your head, fingers interlocked. Press elbows back, (c) arms dangling down, hands relaxed and trailing in the water, (d) hands clasped behind hips, elbows straight. Gently lift arms back to stretch shoulders, but avoid bending trunk and head foward, (e) arms pulling **Oarfish** style (p. 27). Recover arms to the forward SP as leg moves forward; pull arms back as you step, (f) hands clasped and arms held straight out in front. Lean forward as if someone were pulling you by the hands (Fig. 5-1)

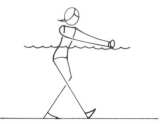

FIGURE 5-1

Step Lively. Briskly walk forward on the balls of your feet, knees slightly bent, toes gripping the pool floor (Fig. 5-2). Use **Step Long** arm positions (a) through (d).

Teeny Tiny Forward Steps. Stand in **chest-deep water.** Now, as you lean forward from the ankles, body straight and on a slant, walk across the pool taking tiny, fast steps on the balls of your feet. Keep stomach pulled in, buttocks muscles tight, knees straight and close together. Use arm positions suggested for **Step Long** except (e) and (f).

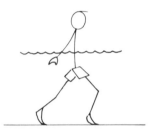

FIGURE 5-2

Lift Knee and Push. Start with arms forward at the surface, palms down. Now, take giant steps forward in three precise stages: (a) lift right knee up to right elbow, foot flexed (Fig. 5-3), (b) straighten knee, pushing heel forward and touching toes to right hand (Fig. 5-4), (c) press leg down landing heel first. Repeat across the pool alternating legs. For a good stretch, pause briefly in the "knee up" position and again when touching toes to fingers. To vary, perform with arms in any **Step Long** positions (a) through (d). Lift knees high and extend legs forward with toes close to the surface.

High Step. Step forward on your right foot and lift your left knee; step on your left foot and lift the right knee. Use giant steps lifting knees high and keeping back erect (Fig. 5-5). Hold hands in either (a) or (b) positions suggested for **Step Long.**

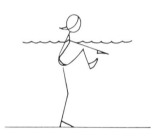

FIGURE 5-3

High Step and Twist. Start with palms on the back of your head, fingers interlocked. Now perform **High Step** and, as you lift the right knee, twist at the waist and swing your left elbow across to meet it. Repeat with the left knee and right elbow (Fig. 5-6). Each time you step forward, straighten up and press your elbows back.

Step—Kick. Step forward on one foot, then swing the other leg forward as though kicking a football. (Lift knee first, then straighten it forward smartly.) Progress across the pool alternating legs. Hold arms out to each side, hands resting on the surface, palms down, or use **Step Long** arm positions (a) through (d).

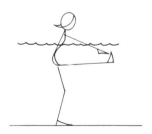

FIGURE 5-4

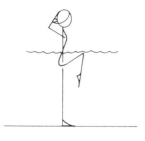

FIGURE 5-5

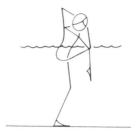

FIGURE 5-6

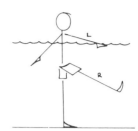

FIGURE 5-7

Poker Walk. Kick your right leg forward, knee straight, foot flexed, then step forward on the right foot, heel first. Repeat with the left leg. Now, add the basic **Penguin** arm movement (p. 30) so that your left leg and right arm swing forward at the same time; then your left arm and right leg (Fig. 5-7). Keep feet flexed and knees, elbows, and fingers stiff like pokers. You also can do this in place.

Kick and Lunge. Kick your right leg forward, knee straight, then step far forward on the right foot to a lunge, Fig. 5-8. (weight on right leg, knee bent; ball of left foot on the floor in back, knee straight). Pause briefly in this position with chest lifted, stomach pulled in. Progress across the pool by alternating legs. Hold hands on hips or stretch arms out to each side, hands just under the surface, palms down. Or, use the following arm movements to add waist, arm, and upper body exercise.

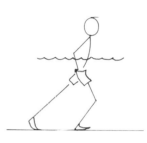

FIGURE 5-8

Clap Down. Do **Kick and Lunge** with arms out to each side and stretched back as far as possible, hands just under the surface, palms down. As you kick up, press arms down and clap hands under your thigh (Fig. 5-9). As you lunge, swing arms up to the SP.

Reach One Arm Forward. Start with arms out to each side, hands just under the surface, palms facing forward. **Kick and Lunge** across the pool; however, as you kick up with the right leg, swing the left arm forward and touch fingers to toes (Fig. 5-10). Lunge forward and press arm back to the SP, then repeat with the left leg and right arm. As you reach forward with one arm, press the other back, and remember to keep hands under the surface.

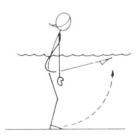

FIGURE 5-9

Reach Both Arms Forward. Start with arms out to each side, hands just under the surface, palms facing forward. Now, **Kick and Lunge** across the pool using the **Booby** arm movement (p. 21). Swing arms forward to touch fingers to toes as you kick up. Swing arms back to the start as you step forward and lunge.

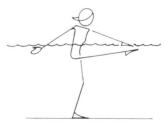

FIGURE 5-10

Reach Up and Over. Kick and Lunge across the pool starting with arms sideward again, hands resting on the surface, this time with palms facing up. As you kick up, swing arms overhead, then down in front to touch fingers to toes (Fig. 5-11). Reverse the arm motion to the SP as you step forward into the lunge. During all sideward arm positions **used in Kick and Lunge,** be sure to stretch arms back as far as possible.

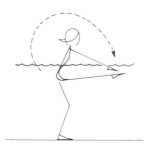

FIGURE 5-11

Kick Across—Lunge Side. Hold your arms in a fixed wide V, hands resting on the surface, palms down. For inner thigh exercise, **Kick and Lunge** across the pool, but kick your leg across to the opposite hand (Fig. 5-12), then lunge diagonally to the side (Fig. 5-13). Keep your trunk facing forward and alternate legs.

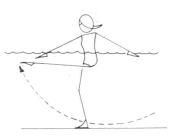

FIGURE 5-12

Step Across. (Adds inner thigh, waist, arm, and upper body exercise.) Walk forward on the balls of your feet, crossing one foot in front of the other. Cross each foot over as far as possible by twisting at the waist. At the same time, swing your arms from side to side in opposition to your forward leg. To do this, start with arms forward in a wide V, hands just under the surface, palms facing one another. Keep elbows straight and maintain the spacing between your hands. Now, swing arms to the right as you step across to the left with the right foot (Fig. 5-14); swing arms left as foot crosses over to the right.

Extended Range. Perform **Step Across** with knees stiff. Swing each leg in an arc, bringing it from behind, out to the side, then step across in front.

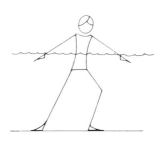

FIGURE 5-13

Lift Knee Across. Perform Step Across but, this time, lift each knee high toward your chest, then swing it across in front before stepping down and across.

Step Backward. Walk backward across the pool, firmly pushing your feet against the floor. Arm position may be either (a) with hands on hips, (b) forward, hands relaxed and trailing in the water, (c) as in **Reverse Oarfish** arm motion (p. 27). Scoop arms forward as you step back, then recover arms to their side SP as other leg moves back for the next step.

Kick Back and Step. To move backward across the pool, step back on one foot, then kick the other leg up to the back. Lean forward slightly to lift it high (Fig. 5-15). Alternate legs. Hold arms forward at the surface, palms down.

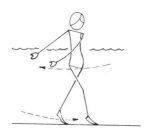

FIGURE 5-14

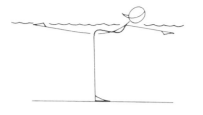

FIGURE 5-15

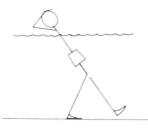

FIGURE 5-16

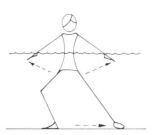

FIGURE 5-17

Teeny Tiny Backward Steps. Lean back while walking backward. Body should be slanted but straight from knees to top of head and with fingers interlocked, palms against the back of your head. Press elbows back and maintain a tight Tuck-in (Fig. 5-16). Next, speed up the action so that you are taking tiny, fast steps while pushing against the floor with your toes. See how far back you can lean without falling over.

Slide Wide to the Side. Walk sideways taking giant steps and bringing feet together with each step (i.e., slide one foot far to the side, then firmly pull the other leg in to meet it). Position hands on hips or hold arms out to each side, hands resting on the surface, palms down. Periodically move in the opposite direction.

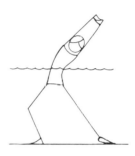

FIGURE 5-18

Lift—Press. Do Slide Wide to the side, but start with arms down at your sides. Lift them sideward to the surface as you slide foot to the side (Fig. 5-17); forcefully press arms down to the SP as you bring feet together.

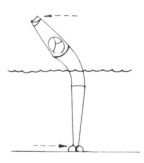

FIGURE 5-19

Slide 'n Arch. For extra waist exercise, do **Slide Wide to the side** with hands clasped overhead, elbows straight, then turn palms to face up. Now, arch your trunk to the left as you slide the left foot sideward (Fig. 5-18); arch to the right as foot slides to meet the left (Fig. 5-19). Keep elbows straight. Reverse the action when stepping to the right.

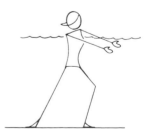

FIGURE 5-20

Reach Side—Swing Across. Start with arms diagonally forward to the left, elbows straight, arms shoulder-width apart and with palms facing one another. Step left foot to the left (Fig. 5-20). Now you're ready to slide right foot to meet the left as you vigorously swing arms across in front to the right (Fig. 5-21). Pause briefly to bend elbows and slide hands toward you, ready to reach out and step again. For easy coordination, repeat to yourself, "1" (reach and step side), "2" (swing arms across and step feet together). Reverse the arm motion when stepping to the right. Remember to keep hands under the surface. To vary, perform with right arm only when stepping to the right (put left hand on your hip); use left arm when stepping left.

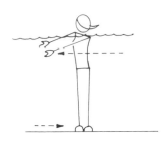

FIGURE 5-21

Circle 'n Slide. This time, swing your arms in a large circle under the surface as you **Slide Wide to the Side.** Start with feet together, arms forward at the surface, palms down with thumbs touching. Slide one foot sideward as you press arms down, back, and up to the side, turning palms to face forward; bring feet together as you scoop arms forward to the start.

Scamper Side. Scamper sideways across the pool taking small, quick steps on the balls of your feet. Bring your feet together with each step. Avoid bouncing by keeping knees stiff, body erect, and shoulders on an even keel. Hold arms either (a) with hands on hips, (b) sideward with hands at the surface, palms down, or (c) down at your sides. Periodically scamper in the opposite direction.

LILY TROTTER

GET SET: Stand in **waist-to-chest-deep water.**

GO: This group shows how to jog, either in place, back and forth across the pool, or at the wall and how to run in waist-high or deep water.

Jog Free. To jog the Aquacises way, lift knees high in a clipped or stacatto fashion. Land on the balls of your feet and roll down to your heels.[9]

1. Jog forward, backward, or in place (a) with hands on hips, (b) hands clasped behind hips, elbows straight, or (c) palms against back of head, fingers interlocked, elbows pressed back.

[9]The Aquacises methods of jogging and running in the water (i.e., the manner in which the feet strike the floor) should not be used on land where they could be stressful to feet and other supporting joints. The reverse is true in the water, thanks to its buoyancy.

2. Jog in place with palms against the back of your head, fingers interlocked. For waist exercise, (a) bend from side to side, bending right as you step on right foot; left as you step on left foot, or (b) twist at the waist and turn shoulders right as you step on left foot; turn left as you step on right.

3. Jog in place while raising and lowering arms as in **Butterflyfish** (p. 26). Lift arms as you step on right foot; press them down as you step on left.

4. Jog forward, backward, or in place using arms in push-pull fashion (push one hand forward as you pull the other back, hands under the surface, fingers curled lightly into fists). Use one arm change for each step.

5. Jog in place with (a) arms down at your sides or (b) arms out to each side, fingers curled into fists. As you jog, rotate arms in circles—one circle for each step.

6. Jog forward, backward, or in place using the basic **Penguin** arm motion (p. 30) or its variation **Double Swing,** with fingers curled into fists. Change arm position once for each step.

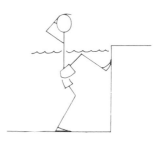

FIGURE 5-22

7. For waist-slimming exercise, jog in place by lifting knees across body. In other words, jog on right foot as you lift left knee up and across to the right; jog on left foot as you lift right knee across. To add stability to your twisting motions, hold arms in a wide V, hands just under the surface, palms facing forward. Try to bring knee to opposite elbow.

8. Jog forward or in place while using the basic **Oarfish** arm movement (p. 27).

9. Jog with arms out to each side, hands at the surface, palms down. This time, lift knees sideward to elbows. Land far to each side to separate feet as much as possible.

Jog at the Wall

1. Stand facing the wall with palms against the back of your head, fingers interlocked, or clasp hands in back of hips, elbows straight. Place one foot halfway up on the wall (Fig. 5-22). (As you progress, strive to bring toes up to surface level.) Now, jog by exchanging the position of your legs. To vary, cross each knee over as in #7 **Jog Free,** touching right foot to the wall at the left; left foot to the wall at the right.

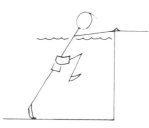

FIGURE 5-23

2. Stand facing the wall about three feet out. Lean forward and hold the ledge with body straight and on a slant. Jog by lifting knees high and landing lightly on your toes (Fig. 5-23). Avoid bouncing—keep shoulders still. To *vary*, use **Jog Free** suggestion #7.

3. Use #2 SP. Keeping feet flexed, jog by lifting heels back as if to kick your backside (Fig. 5-24). Land flatfooted. To vary, perform as suggested but kick heels across in back.

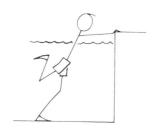

FIGURE 5-24

4. Stand erect, arms' length from the wall and hold the ledge with hands slightly more than shoulder-width apart. This time, jog by lifting knees high to the side (try to lift knees to the level of your elbows, Fig. 5-25). Land on the balls of your feet as far to each side as possible. Use your arms to help lift and support you.

5. Jog from a horizontal position. Keep feet flexed and draw knees under body (Fig. 5-26). Shoot legs back forcefully with a jabbing motion. To vary, use **Jog Free** suggestion #7, rolling to right hip as right knee moves up; then to left hip as right knee straightens and left knee moves up. Bend elbows as necessary for support and balance.

6. Jog while suspended vertically in **water at least chin deep** (Fig. 5-27). Keep feet flexed and straighten knees pushing heels down hard with a jabbing motion. To vary, use **Jog Free** suggestion #7.

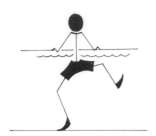

FIGURE 5-25

Note. Aqua-jogging may also be done while holding a kickboard or swim wing in each hand. Keeping head above the surface, you can jog on your side (Fig. 5-28) or, by holding arms sideward, you can jog on your back (Fig. 5-29), front (Fig. 5-30), or vertically. Keep feet flexed and extend legs with a jabbing motion. For front and back versions, perform with body on an angle. Further back, front, or vertical variations may be found under **Jog Free** #7, and by lifting knees sideward to elbows as in #4 above.

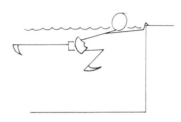

FIGURE 5-26

Toes Up. With hands in any of the positions given in **Jog Free** #1, jog onto your right foot as you lift the left foot forward to the surface. Keep going, changing legs each time. Bend your knees and flex your feet to bring them high (Fig. 5-31). Wow!

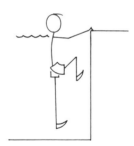

FIGURE 5-27

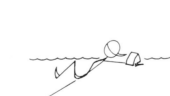

FIGURE 5-29

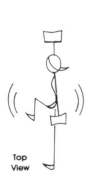

Top
View

FIGURE 5-28

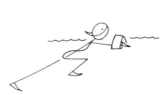

FIGURE 5-30

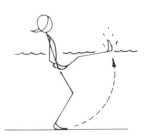

FIGURE 5-31

Pitter—Patter. Stand in **chest-deep water** with arms forward at the surface, palms down. Bend knees to bring water level up to shoulders. Now, jog in place, forward, or backward by briskly lifting right knee to right elbow (Fig. 5-32), left knee to left elbow. Keep shoulders down in the water and avoid bobbing. Land lightly on your toes with your back erect, stomach pulled in. For variety, (a) perform with hands clasped behind hips, elbows straight or (b) hold arms sideward, hands at the surface, palms down. From this position, jog in place by lifting knees sideward to elbows.

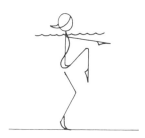

FIGURE 5-32

Run! Run in Aquacises fashion by bounding through the water taking large steps (as if bounding over prickly sea urchins) and covering as much distance as possible with each. Land lightly on the balls of your feet.

1. Run forward pulling arms **Oarfish** style, once for every two steps. (Pull arms back as you step on right foot; move arms forward to the SP as you step on the left.)
2. With elbows straight, run forward circling arms forward, down, back, and overhead in a windmill motion—first one arm, then the other. Plunge arm into the water with each step (Fig. 5-33).
3. Run forward. Use version #2 above, but circle arms simultaneously—one revolution for each two steps. That is, swing arms forward and down as you step on right foot, then swing them back and overhead as you step on the left.
4. Run backward using the reverse of the previous three arm movements.
5. Run forward circling arms, this time as in **Hydra** variation **Double Circle** (p. 32). Inhale as arms move up; exhale as they move sideward and down. Use one complete circle for each four steps. That is, step two times to lift arms, two times to swing them down.
6. Run for joy! When stepping on right foot, fling arms up to a high V (Fig. 5-34); when stepping on left, bend elbows bringing hands down to chest level.

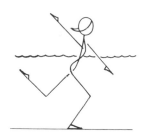

FIGURE 5-33

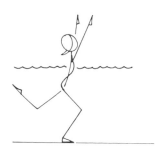

FIGURE 5-34

Smooth Sailing. Stand in **waist-deep water** with arms forward at the surface. Bend knees to bring the water level to your armpits. Now, lean forward and run through the water, propelling yourself along with large steps on the balls of your feet (Fig. 5-35). Avoid bobbing by confining all the action to your legs. To vary, perform with fingers interlocked, palms on the back of your head. Press elbows back.

Run Upstream. Swimmers, run forward in **deep water** while stroking arms **Oarfish** style. Take giant steps as if pedaling a

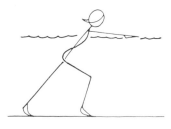

FIGURE 5-35

bicycle. For a greater challenge, omit the arm motion and lean forward slightly with hands on your hips or straight out in front at the surface (Fig. 5-36).

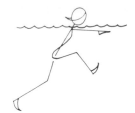

FIGURE 5-36

DOLPHIN

GET SET: Stand in **waist-to-chest-deep water.**

GO: During all **Dolphin** movements, you will jump up and land on both feet simultaneously. Start with small jumps and increase the height as your strength and endurance increase. Nevertheless, thrust upward with vigorous foot and knee action, stretching legs, extending feet, and tightening buttocks as you do; bend knees and Tuck-in as you land. Remember to keep back erect, stomach pulled in.

Pop Up—Feet Together. Jump and land with your feet together. Use any of these arm positions and movements: (a) hands on hips, (b) palms on the back of your head, fingers interlocked, elbows pressed back, (c) arms down at sides, (d) clasp hands overhead, elbows straight. Turn palms to face up, (e) basic **Penguin** arm motion (p. 30) and its variation **Double Swing,** with your fingers curled into fists. Change direction of arms once per jump, (f) **Butterflyfish** arm motion (p. 26). Change direction of arms once per jump. In other words, lift arms sideward as you jump; press arms down as you jump again.

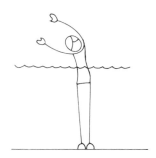

FIGURE 5-37

Open—Close. Jump up and land with feet together. However, at height of jump, quickly open—close legs, separating them either side to side or front to back. Use **Pop Up—Feet Together** arm positions (a) or (b). Or, shoot arms overhead as you jump up, then bend elbows bringing hands to chest as you land.

Pop Overs. Jump up and land with feet together, adding the following waist-firming motion: with arms overhead, jump up and sway arms to the left as you land; jump again and sway arms to the right (Fig. 5-37).

Pop 'n Twist. Jump high and land with a twist at the waist, knees diagonally right. Jump again, landing with knees diagonally left. Perform with feet together or apart. To enhance this waist-firming Aquacise, swing arms from side to side, arms in a wide V, palms facing forward, hands just under the surface. Swing arms right as knees swing left (Fig. 5-38); swing arms left as knees move right. In addition to performing in place, you

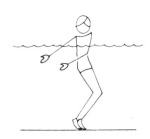

FIGURE 5-38

can pop forward, backward, and to the side. In any case, pop high!

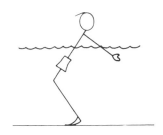

FIGURE 5-39

Pop Backward—Forward. Jump back and forth with feet together. Lean back slightly and press hips forward as you jump forward; then lean forward and press hips back as you jump back. Keep stomach pulled in. Use (a) or (b) arm positions given for **Pop Up—Feet Together.** Also try the **Booby** arm motion (p. 21), pulling arms back as you jump forward (Fig. 5-39); scooping arms forward as you jump back (Fig. 5-40).

Pop Side to Side. With feet together, jump first to one side, then to the other. See how far to each side you can jump. To *vary*, repeat several sequences of one **Pop Backward—Forward** alternating with one **Pop Side to Side.**

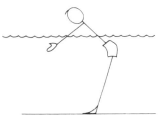

FIGURE 5-40

Pop Up—Feet Apart. Jump up and land keeping feet apart side to side. Use **Pop Up—Feet Together** arm positions (a) through (d).

Close—Open. Jump up and land with feet apart. However, at height of jump, quickly close—open legs. Use **Pop Up—Feet Together** arm positions (a), (b), (d), or (f). When using (f), start with arms sideward and press them down as you close legs, then lift them sideward as you open legs to land. Or, you can clap hands overhead as you close legs; lower them to shoulder level as you land.

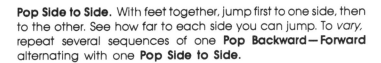

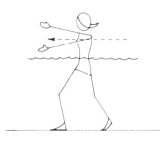

FIGURE 5-41

Swing. (Another super waist trimmer.) Jump up and land keeping feet apart and add the following twisting motion: with arms at shoulder height and separated to a wide V, swing them horizontally from side to side, changing their direction as you land (Fig. 5-41 and 5-42). Feel a vigorous twisting action in your waist. Also try this movement with hands on hips and see how your elbows ripple the water. Start with 6 swings to each side and work up to 12.

Squirt. Stand erect with feet apart in **shoulder-deep water,** arms down at your sides. Pull in your stomach and tighten your buttocks. Now, staying in place, jump up and land first on your toes, then roll down to your heels. Keep your back straight and and knees stiff (like **Spurt,** p. 85, the thrusting action comes entirely from the feet.)

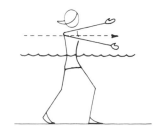

FIGURE 5-42

Flapdoodle. Stand on the balls of your feet in **chest-deep water,** feet apart and with arms sideward, hands just under the surface (or on your hips). Bend knees to submerge shoulders.

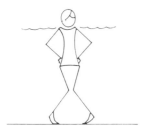

FIGURE 5-43

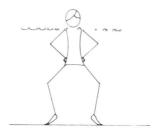

FIGURE 5-44

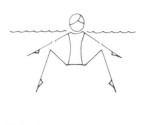

FIGURE 5-45

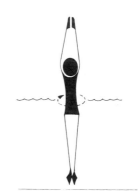

FIGURE 5-46

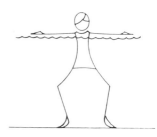

FIGURE 5-47

Now, swing knees together, turning toes in (Fig. 5-43); then swing knees sideward, turning toes out (Fig. 5-44). Perform briskly, lifting feet lightly to change position. Keep shoulders down in the water and avoid bobbing.

Hot Foot. Stand on tiptoe in **shoulder-deep water** with feet far apart. Hold arms sideward, hands just under the surface. Now, rapidly lift knees up to elbows (Fig. 5-45) then push legs down to the start, landing lightly on your toes. Avoid bobbing—keep shoulders down in the water and confine all the action to your legs.

Pop 'n Whirl. Jump up and spin around 180° before landing. Begin and end each jump with arms sideward, feet apart, knees bent and **water at shoulder level** (Fig. 5-46). Jump up and, as you turn, bring feet together and clap hands overhead (Fig. 5-47). Keep body in alignment, with buttocks tucked under and stomach pulled in. To add momentum to your spin, bounce once between each jump.

Flying High. Start with arms at your sides, feet together. Now, jump up and land with feet apart; jump again and land with feet together. As you jump with feet apart, swing arms sideward and clap hands overhead; as you jump with feet together, plunge arms down to the start. (Be sure to press them all the way to your sides.) For a less vigorous arm motion, use the **Butterflyfish** (p. 26).

Pop 'n Cross. Jump up and land with your feet apart side to side (Fig. 5-48). Jump again and land with your right foot crossed in front of the left (Fig. 5-49). As you repeat the sequence, land with alternate feet crossed in front. Hold arms sideward, hands just under the surface, or clasp hands behind hips, elbows straight. In addition, you can choose among **Pop Up—Feet Together** arm positons (a), (b), or (d).

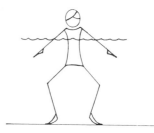

FIGURE 5-48

Jump 'n Lunge. Jump high and land with legs in a lunge position (weight on forward leg, knee bent; ball of opposite foot on floor in back, knee straight). Land each time with the opposite leg forward, exchanging their positions during the jump. Keep chest up and back erect. Use **Pop Up — Feet Together** arm positions (a) through (e). During (e), swing right arm and left leg forward, then left arm and right leg (Fig. 5-50).

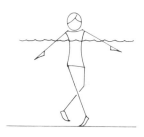

FIGURE 5-49

Scissor Legs. Perform **Jump 'n Lunge,** but keep knees stiff the entire time and use foot action only. Use small jumps, landing lightly on the balls of your feet. Place hands on hips.

Double Time. Squat down in the water with hands on hips. **Jump 'n Lunge** but, this time, omit the jump and change leg position rapidly, skimming feet along the floor. Land lightly on the balls of your feet, keep shoulders down in the water and avoid bobbing. If you like, repeat several sequences alternating between two slow leg changes and four rapid ones.

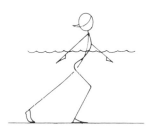

FIGURE 5-50

Pop Forward. Jump up and land, progressing forward during the upward thrust. Jump either with (a) feet together, (b) feet apart side to side, or (c) feet alternately apart then together. Use **Pop Up — Feet Together** arm positions (a) or (b), or pull arms **Oarfish** style (p. 27). Pull arms back as you jump once; recover arms to the forward SP as you jump again. Maintain your Tuck-in so that you land with body in alignment.

Pop Backward. Jump up and land, moving backward with each jump. Use any of the foot and arm positions given for **Pop Forward;** however, use the reverse **Oarfish** motion.

Pop Sideward. With feet together, repeat several sequences of eight jumps to the right with eight to the left. Hold arms out to each side, hands just under the surface, or use **Pop Up — Feet Together** arm positions (a), (b), or (d).

Spurt. Stand in **chest-to-shoulder-deep water** with feet either apart or together. Now, as you lean forward from the ankles, body straight and on a slant, jump forward across the pool as though you were a pogo stick. Keep legs stiff and use lots of foot action to push off (Fig. 5-51). Land on your toes, then roll down to heels. On the up motion, tighten buttocks, stretch legs, and extend feet. The idea is to see how far you can lean without falling over or poking out your backside. Use **Pop Up — Feet Together** arm positions (a), (b), or (c). Or, clasp hands behind hips with elbows straight. Gently lift arms back to stretch shoulders.

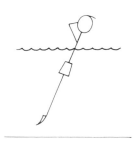

FIGURE 5-51

Kick Up—Pop Forward. To move forward across the pool, first kick one leg forward (Fig. 5-52) then vigorously push off the floor with the supporting foot and bring feet together to land (Fig. 5-53). Repeat several times before kicking the opposite leg, or alternate legs. Either (a) hold arms out to each side, hands just under the surface, (b) place hands on hips, or (c) use arms **Oarfish** style (p. 27). Pull arms back as you jump forward; recover arms to the forward SP as you kick forward. You also can do this movement by kicking and jumping to the side using arm position (a).

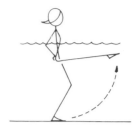

FIGURE 5-52

Bounce on the Wall. To strengthen your hands, arms, trunk and legs, stretch your lower back and legs and, for moderate cardiovascular benefits, face the wall in **water at least chest deep.** Firmly hold the pool rim with hands shoulder-width apart. (Keep hands in this position throughout each movement.) Tuck up knees tightly, stomach pulled in, and brace feet together against the wall (Fig. 6-1). Land in this position after each of these jumping Aquacises (excluding #6):

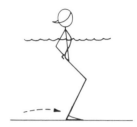

FIGURE 5-53

1. Spring away from the wall, thrusting hips back and straightening knees momentarily (Fig. 5-54). To vary, quickly open—close legs when hips are back and knees are straight. Then bend knees and land.
2. Perform #1 but land with a twist at the waist, bending knees as you land and swinging hips around to one side to touch your backside to the wall. Jump again and swing hips to the wall at the other side.
3. Perform #1 landing with feet alternately on the wall at the right, then on the left.
4. Jump up lightly and land with one knee bent, the other leg extended to the side, knee straight, toes on the wall. Jump again and land with both knees bent in the SP. Repeat to the other side. Or, omit returning to the SP each time and jump side to side alternating legs.
5. Jump up lightly and land with feet apart on the wall (Fig. 5-55). Jump again and slide feet together, landing in the SP.
6. Jump up lightly and extend one leg down and back, straightening knee (Fig. 5-56). Alternate legs.

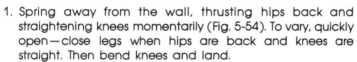

FIGURE 5-54

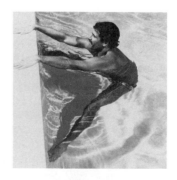

Rise and Shine. Swimmers, for overall stretch and tone, do the following movements in water at least **chest-to-shoulder deep.** Alternately jump high and inhale, then submerge, bringing feet to the floor and exhaling. Stretch legs as you jump up, keeping body in alignment—back erect, buttocks tucked under, stomach pulled in.

FIGURE 5-55

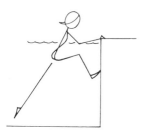

FIGURE 5-56

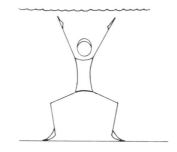

FIGURE 5-57

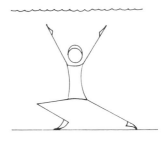

FIGURE 5-58

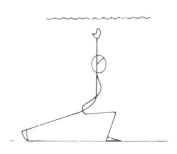

FIGURE 5-59

1. Jump high and land with knees tightly tucked up, feet to-gether (Fig. 7-12). Perform in place or progress forward by rising on a slant. To vary, bring your buttocks and heels to the floor during each submergence and/or at the height of the jump; quickly open—close legs, separating them to the side.
2. Keeping feet apart, jump and land with knees bent outward, (Fig. 5-57). To vary, at height of jump, quickly close—open legs.
3. Jump high, landing with one knee bent, the other leg extended sideward, knee straight (Fig. 5-58). Alternate legs by exchanging their position during the jump.
4. Jump high and land in a deep lunge (Fig. 5-59). Alternate legs by exchanging their position during each jump. To vary, start in a deep lunge, then jump up and quickly "scissors" legs once (knees straight) to land with legs in the SP.

Try the following arm positions and movements for **Rise and Shine:** (a) Clasp hands behind hips, elbows straight. (b) Hold arms forward, palms down. Pull arms down to front of thighs as you thrust upward; lift arms up to the start as you submerge. (c) Hold arms sideward, hands just under the surface, palms down. Pull arms down to your sides as you thrust up (Fig. 5-60); lift arms to the start as you submerge. (d) For **Rise and Shine** #4, use arms **Penguin** style (p. 30) so that you land with the right leg and left arm forward; then the left leg and right arm. For all arm movements, keep elbows straight and press arms forcefully through the water.

SAND HOPPER

GET SET: Stand in **waist-to-chest-deep water.**

GO: When doing **Sand Hopper,** you'll land on one foot at a time instead of both feet simultaneously as in **Dolphin** Aquacises. Keep chest up and stomach pulled in.

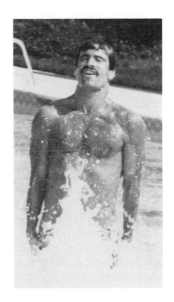

FIGURE 5-60

Forward Hop. Perform this movement in **chest-deep water** by hopping forward on one foot with the other leg raised high in front, knee straight (Fig. 5-61). Firmly push foot against the floor as you thrust up and bring heel to the floor as you land. Hop on one foot halfway across the shallow end of the pool, then change leg position and continue across. Use any of these arm positions: (a) hands on hips, (b) hands clasped behind hips, elbows straight, arms lifted back to stretch shoulders, (c) arms forward, hands resting on the surface, palms down, (d) arms pulling **Oarfish** style (p. 27). Pull arms back as you spring up; recover them to the forward SP as you land. Hop high!

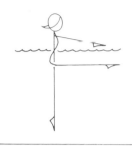

FIGURE 5-61

Hold Your Foot 'n Hop. Lift one knee toward your chest and grasp your toes, one hand on each side of your foot (Fig. 5-62). Now, hop forward on the other foot. Change to the opposite foot periodically. To vary, (a) hop backward or (b) intersperse forward or backward hops with an occasional turn (hop four times to turn 360°). Hop high!

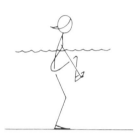

FIGURE 5-62

Bun-ny Hop. Bend your knees until the **water is at shoulder level,** then grasp a "bun" in each hand (as if to sit in your hands). Now, hop onto your right foot as you kick the left foot up, straightening your knee sharply (Fig. 5-63). Then, hop onto the left foot, straightening the right knee. Hop briskly, landing lightly on your toes. Avoid bobbing—keep shoulders down in the water but lift feet as high as possible.

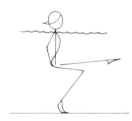

FIGURE 5-63

Hold Your Thigh 'n Hop. Lift your right knee at least to hip level and grasp your thigh with both hands (Fig. 5-64). Now, alternately straighten and bend your knee as you hop in place. Hop once and straighten knee; hop again and bend it. Keep back erect, elbows pointing sideward, and try to hold knee at a constant level as you straighten it. Periodically change to the other leg.

Backward Hop. In **chest-deep water,** lean forward and lift one leg up to the back, knee straight, heel close to the surface (Fig. 5-65). From this position, push your foot against the floor and thrust yourself backward, straightening the forward knee and gliding momentarily (Fig. 5-66). Bend knee as you land. Maintain the forward angle of your trunk, but keep head erect, extended leg high. Alternate legs after every eight hops. Either (a) hold arms forward, hands at the surface or (b) use the reverse **Oarfish** arm movement (p. 27). Scoop arms forward as you rise; recover arms to the forward SP as you land. To vary, repeat several sequences of eight **Forward Hops,** alternating with eight **Backward Hops.** Reverse leg position for each sequence.

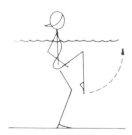

FIGURE 5-64

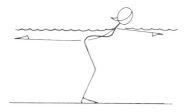

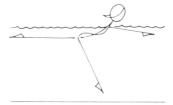

FIGURE 5-65

FIGURE 5-66

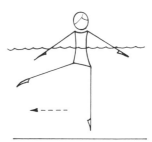

FIGURE 5-67

Sideward Hop. Hop to the *right* with the *right* leg elevated high to the side (Fig. 5-67). Thrust upward vigorously with each push of your foot against the floor. Change legs and repeat to the left side. Hold arms sideward, hands just under the surface.

Sideward Hop—Pump Knee. Hop in place or move to the *left* while vigorously pumping your *left* knee up and down. Keep knee bent and hop once as you lift it (Fig. 5-68); hop again as you press it down behind the supporting leg (Fig. 5-69). Periodically pump right knee and move to the right. Use any of these arm positions: (a) hand on hips, (b) palms on the back of head, fingers interlocked, elbows pressed back, or (c) arms sideward, hands just under the surface. With this position, lift knee to elbow.

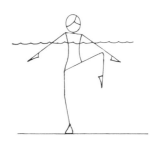

FIGURE 5-68

Make It Snappy. Combine hopping in place with the **Snapper** variation **Snap Side** (p. 65). Hop once as you straighten knee; hop again as you bend it. Place hands on hips or hold arms out to each side, hands just under the surface. (As you straighten knee, lift toes up to fingers.) For variation and extra waist exercise, add a side bend. With hands clasped on top of your head or extended overhead, bend toward knee as it straightens (Fig. 5-70); then bend to the other side as foot swings down in back (Fig. 5-71).

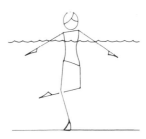

FIGURE 5-69

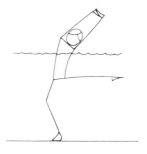

FIGURE 5-70

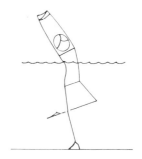

FIGURE 5-71

Hop Kick to the Front. With back erect, hop onto one foot as you kick the other leg forward. Alternate legs, kicking high and lifting toes to the surface. Keep kicking knee straight, but bend supporting knee as you land. Try to stay in one place. Use any of these arm positions: (a) hands on hips, (b) hands clasped behind hips, elbows straight, or (c) to trim the waist, place hands on hips then briskly swing shoulders from side to side, rippling the water with your elbows. Swing right elbow forward as you kick left leg forward; then left elbow and right leg.

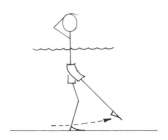

FIGURE 5-72

Scuttle. Hop Kick to the Front but keep your kick low and scuttle forward across the pool. Place hands on hips or on top of head, fingers interlocked, elbows pressed back (Fig. 5-72).

Hop Kick Your Hands. Hold your arms forward with hands at the surface. Now, hop onto one foot as you kick the other leg forward (Fig. 5-73). Continue to hop and kick, changing legs each time. Try to kick up to your hands, foot extended. Keep the kicking knee straight, but bend the supporting knee as you land.

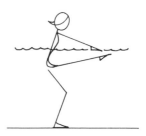

FIGURE 5-73

Hop Kick 'n Tilt. Do **Hop Kick to the Front** while leaning far back. Body should be straight but on a slant. See how far back you can lean without losing your balance. This Aquacise will move you backward. Either (a) place hands on hips, (b) hold arms sideward, hands just under the surface, or (c) for the greatest challenge, place palms against the back of your head, fingers interlocked, elbows pressed back (Fig. 5-74). To vary, repeat several sequences of six of this movement with six **Hop Kick Your Hands.** Afterward, walk slowly to catch your breath—then, do it again!

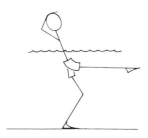

FIGURE 5-74

Hop Kick to the Back. Lean forward and hop onto one foot as you kick the other leg high to the back. Alternate legs, keeping knee of kicking leg straight. Either (a) hold arms forward at the surface, palms down, (b) hold onto the pool ledge (Fig. 5-75), (c) place hands on hips, or (d) interlock fingers and place palms on the back of your head, elbows pressed back. To vary, repeat several sequences of eight **Hop Kick to the Front** with eight to the back. Hold arms as in (c) or (d) above.

Hop Kick Your Backside. Hop onto one foot as you kick the other foot toward your buttocks, bending knee sharply (Fig. 5-76). Perform in place or progress forward across the pool while alternating legs. Keep back erect, stomach pulled in, and hop high! You can do them straight with hands on hips or with a twist—hands either behind your head or on your hips.

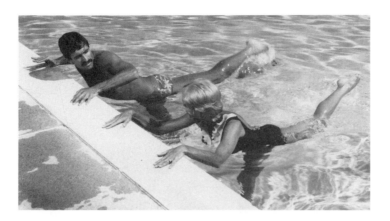

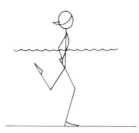

FIGURE 5-76

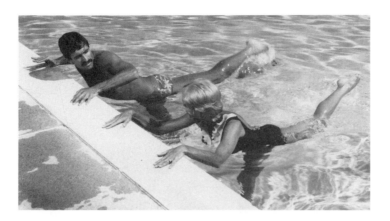

FIGURE 5-75

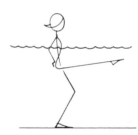

Twist right when hopping on right foot; twist left when hopping on left.

Rock Forward and Back. Start with the right leg forward, knee straight (Fig. 5-77). Now, spring up and over an imaginary barrel, landing on your right foot, knee bent, left leg stretched up to the back (Fig. 5-78). Next, hop back on the left foot, bending knee as you kick right leg forward to the SP. After several repetitions, perform with the left leg forward. Be sure to hop forward and back as far as possible to maintain maximum distance between feet. Either (a) place hands on hips or (b) use the **Booby** arm movement (p. 21). Pull arms back as you spring forward, then scoop arms forward as you spring back. To vary, progress forward across the pool. Spring forward, covering as much distance as possible, then draw other foot forward as you rock back on it. Pull arms back vigorously as you spring forward as in (b) above. Midway across the pool, reverse leg position.

Rock Side to Side. Starting with feet apart side to side, hop from one foot to the other in an energetic rocking motion. Hop far to each side to maintain maximum distance between feet and, as you land, bend your supporting knee and lift the other leg high to the side (Fig. 5-79). Keep back erect, buttocks tucked under. Do this either (a) with hands on hips, (b) arms out to each side, hands at the surface. Try to kick up to hands, or (c) clasp hands overhead and bend side to side in the direction of the elevated leg.

Hippety-Hop. Skip like you did as a little kid. Remember? Just step forward on your right foot, then give a little hop and

FIGURE 5-77

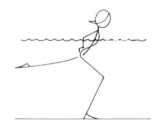

FIGURE 5-78

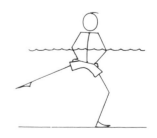

FIGURE 5-79

repeat with the left foot. As you move along, keep your back erect, lift your knees high, and spring up with force. Either (a) place hands on hips, (b) interlock fingers and place palms against the back of your head, or (c) hold arms out to each side and swing them in a carefree manner, skimming hands through the surface.

Variations:

1. Run and skip two widths of the pool using three running steps alternating with two skips; or skip·two and run four (steps).
2. Run two widths of the pool then skip two widths, skipping for height (thrust upward vigorously). Repeat the sequence, skipping for distance. (Cover as much distance as possible with each skip.)

Leap for Joy! Stand in **chest-deep water,** right leg forward, toes close to the surface. Lean forward reaching toward right foot (Fig. 5-73). Now, using the **Oarfish** arm motion, leap forward onto the right foot as you pull arms back. Repeat by recovering arms to the forward SP as you lift left leg forward, ready to leap onto the left foot. As you leap, stretch legs far apart and lift chest (Fig. 5-80). As you land, bring your heel to the floor and stretch the other leg back (Fig. 5-81). Perform across one or more widths of the pool, leaping either for height (spring over an imaginary school of fish) or for distance (cover as much distance as possible with each leap). This also is fun while holding hand paddles and, if you are a swimmer, wearing a swim wing on each ankle to give added impetus to your soaring action.

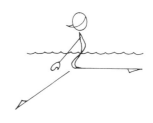

FIGURE 5-80

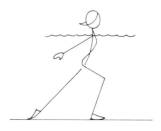

FIGURE 5-81

Variations:

1. Run and leap two widths of the pool using two running steps alternating with one leap. Strive for height when leaping. Or you can run three and leap two.
2. Skip and leap four widths of the pool by skipping two widths, then leaping two widths. Skip for height and leap for distance.

SALMON

GET SET: Hold onto the pool ledge in the manner given for each Aquacise below.

GO: Kick your legs using any one or a combination of these movements. Change from one to the other as desired. Be sure to relax muscles of neck and shoulders and don't hold your breath.

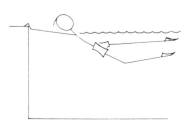

FIGURE 5-82

Just for Kicks. (Page 140 offers suggestions for improving your flutter kick.)

1. Flutter kick on your front, head out of the water, and holding the ledge as shown in Fig. 5-82.
2. Time your flutter kicking. Simply kick slowly as you count to 30 (or use a pace clock on the pool wall and time yourself for ½ minute); then kick briskly for another 30 counts. Repeat several times. As you practice, try to increase the duration of the brisk kick to one minute or more. Breast stroke kick may be substituted for the slow flutter kick if desired, or you can stand close to the wall and jog at an easy pace.
3. Flutter kick from a vertical position by holding the ledge with one side toward the wall, elbow straight or braced against the wall. Hold the other arm sideward, hand at the surface (Fig. 5-83). Periodically kick with other side toward the wall.
4. Flutter kick while lying on one side and holding the ledge in either position shown in Fig. 4-71 or Fig. 5-84. Periodically turn to the other side.
5. Flutter kick on your back from any of the positions shown in Figs. 4-104, 4-105, or 4-108. Keep knees under the water but let toes "bubble" the surface.
6. Push away from the wall, then kick forward (Method #1). To do this, first assume the position shown in Fig. 5-84, with heels close to the surface, legs straight and together. Now, inhale and put your face down in the water as you vigorously shove yourself backward away from the wall. As momentum diminishes, flutter kick forward to the wall. Repeat several times by catching a quick breath just before shoving off.
7. Push away from the wall, then flutter kick forward (Method #2). See Fig. 5-85 for the SP. From there, extend legs to the surface in back (Fig. 5-84). Next, straighten elbows and push backward away from the wall. When momentum diminishes, kick forward then grasp the ledge and pull smoothly to the tucked SP. Keep head up the entire time.

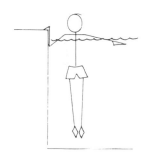

FIGURE 5-83

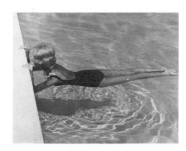

FIGURE 5-84

Lickety-Split. A scissors split motion not to be confused with the scissors kick used in the side stroke. During **Lickety-Split,** the knees are kept straight.

1. Lie on one side and hold the pool ledge with the upper hand while pressing palm of lower hand against the wall,

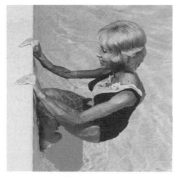

FIGURE 5-85

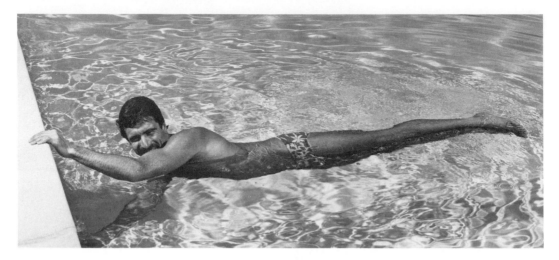

FIGURE 5-86

fingers pointing down (Fig. 5-86). Tuck-in and stretch/tense legs. Now, swing legs forward and backward in a rapid scissors motion. Separate legs as far as possible and swing them parallel to the surface. Keep knees stiff and feet extended. Repeat on the other side.

2. Scissors your legs from a vertical position, one side toward the wall, in **water at least chin deep.** With the right side toward the wall, hold the pool rim with elbow either straight or braced against the wall (Fig. 5-83). Extend the right arm sideward. Stretch/tense legs as you swing them back and forth with feet extended or flexed. Then, repeat with other side toward wall.

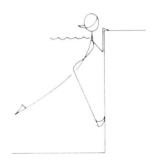

FIGURE 5-87

3. Scissors your legs from a vertical position, this time facing the wall. In **water at least chin deep,** hold the ledge with (a) elbows straight, (b) elbows braced against the wall (Fig. 5-87), or (c) arms resting on the deck, one on top of the other, and with elbows bent, chin resting on hands. Brace the toes of one foot against the wall and extend the other leg back. Now, swing your legs back and forth scissors fashion, moving one leg forward as you move the other back. Stretch legs as you firmly push them through the water and bring toes to the wall with each forward movement. To vary, (a) perform with elbows straight and bring sole of foot high on the wall (Fig. 6-29) or (b) twist at the waist swinging your leg across in front to touch toes to the wall.

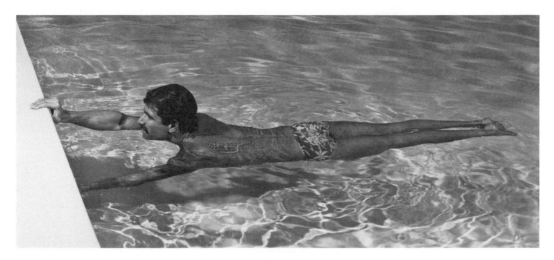

FIGURE 5-88

V-Split and Cross. Lie front down and hold the pool ledge either (a) with elbows braced against the wall as shown in Fig. 5-84 or (b) with upper hand while pressing palm of lower hand against the wall, fingers pointing down (Fig. 5-88). Now, briskly open legs sideward to a V-split, then close them, crossing at the angles (first right over left, then left over right, etc.) Stretch legs, extend feet, and lift heels. To vary, (a) perform with body on a slat (Fig. 5-89) for less stress to the lower back, or (b) with body vertical and facing the wall, with elbows straight or braced against the wall.

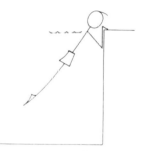

FIGURE 5-89

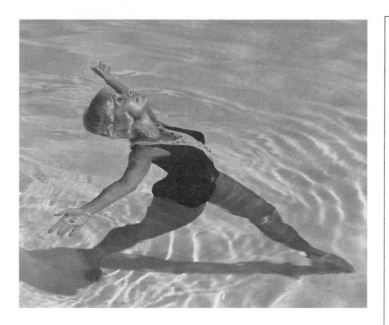

Chapter 6
STRETCHAWAY AQUACISES

Stretchaway Aquacises tone the body, relieve tension, and loosen tight muscles resulting from stress and inactivity. While many Aquacises improve joint and muscle elasticity, these movements provide more variety and a different range of motion. Most are performed slowly, using the pool ledge and the water's buoyancy for support. However two other groups of Stretchaways in this chapter include (1) posture-control Aquacises stressing the Tuck-in position (**Humpback** through **Pufferfish**) and (2) stretching movements using floating devices for support (**Feather Duster** group).

Every fitness program should include some stretching to develop the suppleness needed to move easily and gracefully. Besides, a supple body develops fewer aches and pains and is less prone to action injuries. Notwithstanding pre-exercise warm-ups, which may include some easy stretching movements, efforts to increase flexibility are best done when inner body temperature has been raised by other, more vigorous exercises. Therefore, save Stretchaway movements until the end of the session to also avoid breaking the momentum of your workout and diminishing its cardiovascular benefits.

Begin each Stretchaway Aquacise by easing into position. As you repeat the movement, gradually extend the stretch to your maximum. Over time, continue to push your maximum higher. Don't bounce vigorously into maximum-stretch positions because this can produce a stretch-reflex reaction in which the muscles being stretched contract

Stretchaway Aquacises

PIKE (p. 99)
   Bend and Unbend
   Bend—Swing—Bend
   Swing Down and Up
   Swing 'n Touch
SHRIMP (p. 100)
   Hold the Ledge
   Clasp Hands Behind Head
   Lie Back, Arms Sideward
MUDSKIPPER (p. 101)
   Basic Movement
   Bounce Heel Down
   Add a Twist
FALLFISH (p. 102)
   Chest Forward—Hips Back
   Left—Right Side Swing
   Body Circles
   Fall Side, Feet Together
   Fall Side, Knee Side
   Fall Side, Feet Apart
URCHIN (p. 104)
   Basic Movement
   Bend Knees Alternately
   Footwork
   Step Out
PETTICOAT FISH (p. 105)
   Basic Movement
PUMPKINSEED (p. 106)
   Basic Movement
SEA FAN (p. 106)
   Basic Movement
LADY OF THE WATERS (p. 106)
   Basic Movement
   Side Stretch
TIP-UP (p. 107)
   Basic Movement
   Two Choices
SEA CUCUMBER (p. 107)
   Basic Movement
SEA WHIP (p. 108)
   Basic Movement
   Pause and Lift

Pause—Swing One
Pause—Swing Two
NUDIBRANCH (p. 109)
   Basic Movement
   Go Easy
   Two Choices
GOBY (p. 110)
   Basic Movement
HUMPBACK (p. 110)
   Basic Movement
CLINGFISH (p. 111)
   Basic Movement
   Elbows Up
   Fancy Clingfish (Shallow Water)
   Fancy Clingfish (Deep Water)
FLATFISH (p. 112)
   Basic Movement
OYSTER (p. 112)
   Basic Movement
ARCHERFISH (p. 113)
   Touch Back—Chest Up
   Sit Down—Stand Up
   Chest Up—Backside Up
SPINY LOBSTER (p. 114)
   Basic Movement
STICKLEBACK (p. 114)
   Basic Movement
PUFFERFISH (p. 115)
   Basic Movement
   Lift Leg and Return
   Lift Leg and Hold
FEATHER DUSTER (p. 116)
   Pause 'n Stretch
   One Up
   Split to V—Pike—Press Down
   Swing Down and Cross
   Giant Steps
   Twist 'n Step
   Hip Ahoy
   Chug
   Scissors
   Swivel

Tuck—Tip
Pike—Arch
Tuck—Tip—Extend
Split—Tip
Frog Knees to High V-Split
Frog Knees 'n Swing
Arc Side to Side
Tuck—Extend Side

instead. On the other hand, movements like the **Pike, Fallfish, Mudskipper, Petticoat Fish,** and **Urchin** are also fun to do more energetically, but only after a good warm-up.

Unless instructed otherwise, start with 8 repetitions of each of your chosen Stretchaway Aquacises and work up to 15.

PIKE

Stretches your back and the back of your legs. All movements in this group, except Bend and Unbend, stretch the trunk laterally.

GET SET: Face the wall and hold the pool rim with hands shoulder-width apart or hold the ladder bars.

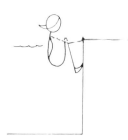

FIGURE 6-1

GO: Use these as separate Aquacises or combine several into a sequence by repeating each a few times before moving to the next.

Bend and Unbend. First, get into the "bend" position. Crouch down in the water and bring your feet up on the wall in front, feet together, knees tucked up tightly (Fig. 6-1). Now, "unbend" to the pike position by slowly straightening your elbows and knees at the same time. As you do, pull in your stomach hard and gently press your heels toward the wall (Fig. 6-2). When knees are straight, your face may be in or out of the

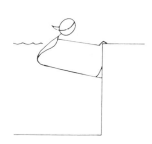

FIGURE 6-2

water (Fig. 6-3). Place feet as high on the wall as flexibility permits. (The higher they are, the greater the stretch, so go easy at first.)

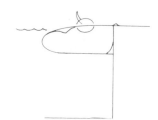

Bend—Swing—Bend. Start in the "bend" position. Now, straighten your knees as you swing your hips to the left. (Pivot on the balls of your feet and lift hips above the surface, Fig. 6-4.) Then bend knees, return to the start, and repeat to the right. For a change, bend and unbend knees several times with hips over to the side.

FIGURE 6-3

Swing Down and Up. Start in the "unbend" position, but with feet midway up the wall. Now, with elbows and knees straight, swing your hips down then up to the other side like a clock's pendulum. Pivot on the balls of your feet, keeping heels close to the wall.

Swing 'n Touch. Start in the "unbend" position. Now, swing hips over to the right side, then bend knees and touch your backside to the wall. Straighten knees, then reverse the motion by swinging hips left before bending knees and touching backside to the wall at the left.

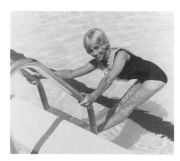

SHRIMP

Strengthens muscles of the abdomen and back of legs

FIGURE 6-4

GET SET: Either hold the pool rim with both hands about shoulder-width apart and walk your feet up the wall into position, or hold on with one hand and swing your legs up. When in position, your legs should be together with lower legs on the deck, your buttocks against the wall, and your hands gripping the rim close to your knees (Fig. 6-5). Adjust the angle of your trunk to bring your head above the water or rest your head on the surface. Pull in your stomach strongly and maintain position by pressing heels down against pool deck.

GO: Begin with the first two, and the easiest, movements. Exhale as you bend forward, inhale as you lie back. Start with 8 and gradually work up to 20 repetitions.

Hold the Ledge

1. With hands in the **Get Set** position, raise your trunk to bring chest close to thighs. Hold momentarily, then slowly return to the start.

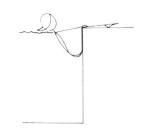

FIGURE 6-5

2. Starting from the **Get Set** position, swing your trunk from side to side.

Clasp Hands Behind Head

1. Start with hands clasped behind your head (elbows pressed back), elbows and head above the surface or resting on It. Now, raise your trunk bringing elbows forward to clasp knees (Fig. 6-6). Slowly return to the start. To avoid neck strain, don't pull your head forward.
2. This time, raise up crossing left elbow over to touch right knee. Return to the start and repeat with the right elbow and left knee.
3. Swing your trunk from side to side touching right elbow to the wall at the right, then left elbow to the wall at the left.

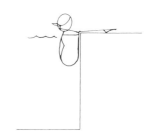

FIGURE 6-6

Lie Back, Arms Sideward

1. Begin with the back of your head and arms resting on the surface, arms sideward, palms facing up. Now, swing your arms back through the surface (Fig. 6-7), then raise up as you swing them overhead and down to touch hands to feet (Fig. 6-8). Reverse the motion back to the start.
2. With arms sideward as in #1, raise your trunk, swinging right arm across to touch left foot. Return to the start, then repeat with the left arm and right foot.
3. Begin as in #1, but swing your trunk from side to side, touching fingers to the wall at each side. Reach far to the side.

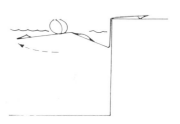

FIGURE 6-7

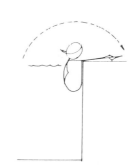

MUDSKIPPER

Firms abdomen, increases flexibility of hips and hamstrings

FIGURE 6-8

GET SET: In **chest-deep water,** stand on the balls of your feet facing the wall about three feet out. Lean forward and hold the pool rim with hands shoulder-width apart. Move your right leg forward, knee bent, to bring toes to the wall in front (Fig. 6-9). Pull in your stomach.

GO: Switch the position of your legs in a smooth continuous motion. To get there, bend both knees high toward your chest, then move legs into position as far apart as possible (right leg back, left forward). During the switch, keep upper body still to avoid bobbing. As you progress, gradually extend the stretch

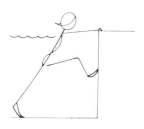

FIGURE 6-9

so that your forward leg is straight with the sole of your foot high on the wall, toes at the surface. Alternate legs.

VARIATIONS:

Bounce Heel Down. To stretch your calf and Achilles' tendon, bounce the heel of your back foot toward the floor. From the **Get Set** position, using left foot action only, bounce up lightly, then press heel down as you land. Bounce three times keeping left knee straight, right foot on the wall. Switch leg position and repeat the sequence several times. In the beginning, bounce gently to avoid overstretching.

Add a Twist. As you bend knees to switch leg position during the basic movement, twist at the waist turning knees right; then place left foot on the wall to the right, right foot across in back (Fig. 6-10). Alternate sides.

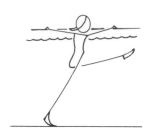

FIGURE 6-10

FALLFISH

Stretches and strengthens all trunk muscles. Strengthens arms and shoulders

GET SET: In **waist-to-chest-deep water,** stand on the balls of your feet facing the wall about three feet out. Lean forward and hold the ledge with hands slightly more than shoulder width apart. Pull in your stomach and tighten your buttocks. Your body should be straight and on a slant.

GO: Use any of the following Aquacises separately or combine them into a sequence by repeating each two or more times before moving to the next. Inhale as body moves forward; exhale as hips move back.

Chest Forward—Hips Back. Bend your elbows and bring your chest close to the wall, keeping elbows high (Fig. 6-11). Next, straighten elbows and press hips back. As you do, pull in your stomach even more, round your back, and tip your head forward (Fig. 6-12). Straighten up, then repeat.

Left—Right Side Swing. Bend your elbows and swing your left side toward the wall, keeping left elbow high to stretch your left side (Fig. 6-13). Next, face the wall as you bend forward and straighten your elbows. At the same time, press your hips back

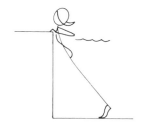

FIGURE 6-11

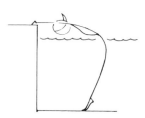

FIGURE 6-12

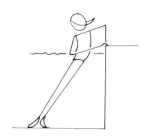

FIGURE 6-13

and pull in your stomach extra hard (Fig. 6-14). Stand upright again, then use the reverse action to bring your right side toward the wall. For extra arm benefits, pull forward and push back vigorously.

Body Circles. Starting in the **Get Set** position, swing your trunk in a circular motion. Bend elbows as you circle forward; straighten them as you circle around to the hips-back position (Fig. 6-14). Stand upright again, then repeat several times in each direction or alternate direction. As you fall foward, tighten your buttocks and pull in your stomach even more to support your lower back. Avoid turning hips and keep your front facing the wall.

Fall Side, Feet Together. This time, **Get Set** by standing erect about a foot from the wall. Now, let your body fall to the right until your shoulders are submerged (Fig. 6-15). Next, give a little push with your hands to right yourself and either (1) fall to the left or (2) push your hips back (Fig. 6-14) then stand upright and fall to the left.

Fall Side, Knee Side. Perform **Fall Side, Feet Together** as suggested, but with one knee bent to the side, foot extended, toes touching the inside of your supporting knee (Fig. 6-16). Press knee outward and fall from side to side omitting hips-back position.

Fall Side, Feet Apart. Stand erect about a foot from the wall with your left leg sideward, foot extended, knee cap facing up. Now, fall to the right keeping leg high (Fig. 6-17) or even lift foot above the surface. Give a little push with your hands to right yourself, then fall to the left until your toes touch the floor far to the side (Fig. 6-18). Lift leg sideward as you pull up to the SP and repeat the entire motion several times before changing

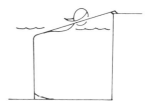

FIGURE 6-14

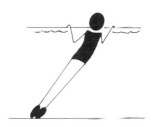

FIGURE 6-15

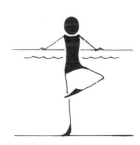

FIGURE 6-16

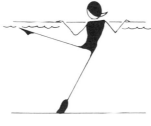

FIGURE 6-17

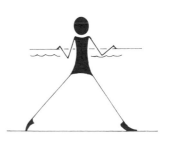

FIGURE 6-18

legs. Constantly stretch your left leg sideward, as if being pulled by the toes, to keep legs in a fixed, wide V-split, both knees straight.

Remember. During the three preceding Aquacises: (1) Keep your front facing the wall. (2) Stand on the balls of your feet. (3) Tighten buttocks and pull in your stomach. (4) As you fall to the side, slide hands along the ledge as necessary to accommodate your changing position. (5) Inhale as you fall; exhale as you stand upright.

URCHIN

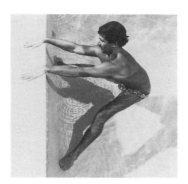

Stretches inner thighs, back of legs, and lower back. Strengthens arms, shoulders, and upper body.

GET SET: Face the wall and hold the pool rim with hands shoulder-width apart. Tuck up knees and place feet side by side on the wall (Fig. 6-1).

GO: Slide your left foot sideward to maximum stretch (Fig. 6-19). Hold the stretch for a slow count of four. Then, keeping knees straight, "walk" your feet zig-zag fashion on the wall to bring them together (i.e., alternately lift toes and pivot on heels to turn toes in; then lift heels and pivot on balls of feet to turn toes out). Lastly, tuck up knees to the SP, then repeat the sequence several times, alternating sides.

FIGURE 6-19

REMEMBER: (1) Move hands along the rim as necessary to accommodate your changing position. (2) When legs are in maximum-stretch position, feet should be slightly higher than hips, flat against the wall, and turned out 45°. (3) Pull in your stomach.

VARIATIONS:

Bend Knees Alternately. From the maximum-stretch position, shift your weight from side to side (shift to the right and bend right knee; then to the left bending the left knee, Fig. 6-20). Keep feet in place, heels on the wall, and bend knee directly over foot. Feel a strong stretch in inner thighs.

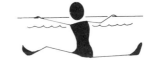

Footwork. From maximum-stretch position, alternately bend and straighten the right knee several times. Each time your knee straightens, tense your leg and flex your right foot (lift toes

FIGURE 6-20

from the wall while keeping heel in place). Feel a stretch in your calf. Repeat with the left leg.

Step Out. From the SP, reach your left foot to the side and step on the wall, bending your left knee. At the same time, move your left hand along the rim to the left to bring hands slightly more than shoulder-width apart. Push foot and hand back to the start and repeat to the right with the right hand and foot. Continue by alternating sides and stepping far to each side.

PETTICOAT FISH

Increases flexibility of hip joints and firms hips, buttocks, and thighs

GET SET: Stand facing the wall in **waist-to-chest-deep water** with your feet together. Rest your hands on the ledge in front and pull in your stomach.

GO: Do these movements with precision and in sequence: (1) Lift your leg as high as possible to the side, knee cap facing forward. (2) Rotate your leg outward to turn your knee cap up. (3) Lift your leg higher. (4) Press leg down to the start. After several repetitions, perform with the other leg. May be done slowly at first; later with vigor.

REMEMBER: (1) Keep hips facing forward by moving only from the hip joint. (2) As you turn knee cap up, tuck your buttocks under. (3) Stretch/tense your working leg from thigh to extended foot. (4) For easy coordination, repeat to yourself, "Lift, rotate, lift, lower."

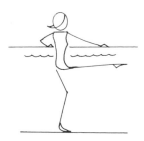

FIGURE 6-21

PUMPKINSEED

Firms buttocks; stretches hip joints

GET SET: Stand facing the wall in **waist-to-chest-deep water,** hands on the ledge shoulder-width apart. Turn hips to the right and lift your right leg forward (Fig. 6-21).

GO: Keeping right leg elevated, turn your trunk to face left (rotate at the hip joint and turn until right leg is extended back). Now, with hands in place, let your weight fall back slightly while stretching your leg back as if being pulled by the toes (Fig. 6-22). Pull yourself upright again, then reverse the rotation and turn to the SP. Repeat several times, then perform with the left leg.

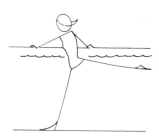

FIGURE 6-22

REMEMBER: (1) Constantly and vigorously stretch/tense your extended leg. As you turn left, feel the action strongly in your right waist, hip, and buttock. (2) Keep back erect, stomach pulled in. (3) Inhale as you turn away from extended leg; exhale as you turn back to the start. (4) Extend leg low at first, but strive for greater heights.

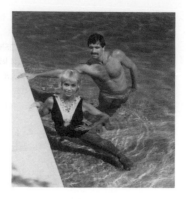

FIGURE 6-23

SEA FAN

Stretches trunk laterally; firms waist, supporting arm, and shoulder

GET SET: Stand in **waist-to-chest-deep water** with your right side about a foot from the wall. Hold onto the pool rim or a ladder bar with your right hand and put your left hand on your hip.

GO: Shove your hips out to the side as you straighten your right arm and arch to the right. Next, pull your hips toward the wall and arch to the left. (Fig. 6-23 shows both positions.) Keep stomach pulled in, buttocks muscles tight. Inhale as hips move out; exhale as they move in toward the wall.

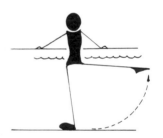

FIGURE 6-24

LADY OF THE WATERS

Increases flexibility of hip joints and firms hips, buttocks, and thighs

GET SET: Stand facing the wall with feet together in **waist-to-chest-deep water.** Rest your hands on the ledge and pull in your stomach.

GO: Kick your right leg high to the side (Fig. 6-24), then reach far to the side with your right foot and step into a side lunge (Fig. 6-25). Kick high to the side again, then press leg down to the start. Repeat several times before changing legs or alternate legs.

REMEMBER: (1) Kick with leg rotated outward to turn knee cap up. (2) Allow your body to lean into the lunge, but maintain a straight back. (3) In the lunge position, bend knee directly over foot. (4) Push hard against the pool floor with the foot of your working leg as you kick up to return to the start. (5) Keep hips facing the wall, stomach pulled in. (6) Inhale as you kick and lunge; exhale as you return to the start.

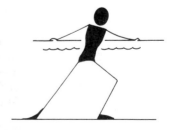

FIGURE 6-25

VARIATION:

Side Stretch. Perform the basic movement. However, as you lunge to the right, swing your left arm overhead and stretch to the right (Fig. 6-26). Bring your left hand back to the ledge as you return to the SP. Be sure to bend directly to the side with elbow on a line with your ear. Repeat to the left, swinging right arm overhead.

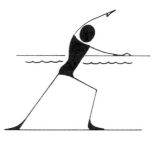

FIGURE 6-26

TIP-UP

Strengthens lower back and buttocks; stretches waist

GET SET: Stand facing the wall in **waist-to-chest-deep water** and hold the ledge with hands far apart.

GO: Tip your trunk forward from the hips and lift the left leg up to the back. Then pivot on the right foot and turn your body as you swing your leg toward the wall at the right, knee straight or bent (Fig. 6-27). Reverse the motion back to the start. Stand upright again and repeat, alternating legs. Swing your leg with toes close to the surface. Follow this Aquacise with the "unbend" position of **Pike** to stretch your back.

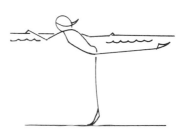

FIGURE 6-27

VARIATIONS:

Two Choices. (1) Omit bringing leg down to the start each time. Instead, substitute a hop (when leg is back) to change from one to the other or (2) try **Tip-Up** while suspended at the wall in deep water. Brace supporting foot low on the wall as shown in Fig. 4-97.

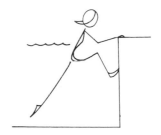

FIGURE 6-28

SEA CUCUMBER

Stretches legs; firms buttocks, arms and shoulders

GET SET: Face the wall in **shoulder-deep water** and hold the rim with hands shoulder-width apart. Brace one foot on the wall in front, knee bent. Stretch the other leg back, with knee straight, foot extended (Fig. 6-28). Next, bend elbows and pull yourself forward touching knee to the wall.

GO: Straighten elbows and knee at the same time, pressing your heel toward the wall (Fig. 6-29). Repeat several times

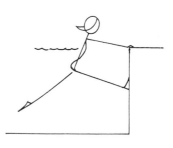

FIGURE 6-29

before reversing leg position. As you bend and straighten, keep your head erect, pull in your stomach, and stretch/lift your extended leg.

SEA WHIP

Stretches trunk and legs; firms arms, shoulders, abdomen, lower back, and buttocks

GET SET: Position yourself at the wall as shown in Fig. 6-30, legs together, shins against the wall, and **water at shoulder level.**

GO: Perform these movements in sequence: (1) Lean forward and brace elbows against the wall as you press legs back to the surface (Fig. 6-31). (2) Straighten elbows and stretch momentarily, Fig. 6-32. (3) Return to the SP in one smooth motion by bending elbows, hips, and knees at the same time.

REMEMBER: (1) When moving into the extended position in Fig. 6-32, stretch legs, tighten buttocks, and lift heels. (2) Just prior to returning to the start, pull in your stomach even more. (3) Inhale as body extends; exhale as legs move forward.

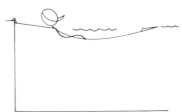

FIGURE 6-30

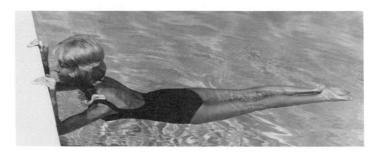

FIGURE 6-31

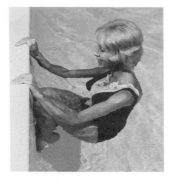

FIGURE 6-32

VARIATIONS:

Pause and Lift. Perform the basic movement, but stop for a slow count of eight in the position shown in Fig. 6-31 while tightening buttocks and lifting heels.

Pause—Swing One. Perform the basic movement, but stop in the extended position (Fig. 6-32) while you swing the right leg forward toward the wall, then back. Repeat with the left leg. For leverage, you can brace left elbow against the wall as right leg moves forward; right elbow when left leg moves forward. Straighten elbow as leg moves back. Keep both legs stretched and close to the surface. To vary, (a) repeat several times before changing to the opposite leg, or swing each leg forward and back once, then bend knees and return to the SP before repeating the sequence.

Pause—Swing Two. Perform the basic movement, but stop in the position shown in Fig. 6-31. Next, straighten elbows as you separate legs and swing feet forward to the wall, legs in a wide V-split (Fig. 6-33). Reverse the motion by bending elbows and swinging legs together in back. Stretch and tense legs and keep them as close to the surface as possible.

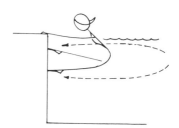

FIGURE 6-33

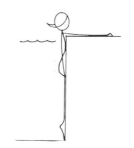

FIGURE 6-34

NUDIBRANCH

Stretches front of body from head to toe; strengthens and firms back, buttocks, and back of thighs

GET SET: In **water at least shoulder deep,** press the front of your body and legs flat against the wall, with arms resting on the deck, elbows straight, edge of pool rim under armpits (Fig. 6-34). Tuck-in tightly and stretch legs with feet extended and together.

GO: Swing your legs away from the wall, lifting heels to the surface in back (Fig. 6-35). Hold the position for a slow count of eight then reverse the action, pressing legs down to the start. To make this movement easier, do it with your knees bent or use the first variation below.

REMEMBER: (1) Gradually "peel" away from the wall beginning with your feet, then your thighs, abdomen, and finally, your rib cage. Reverse the sequence to return to the start. (2) To help lift legs, tighten buttocks and inhale; exhale to help lower legs. (3) Avoid craning your neck—keep head erect. (4) Follow **Nudibranch** with the "unbend" position of **Pike** to stretch back muscles.

VARIATIONS:

Go Easy. For the easiest version of **Nudibranch,** start by holding the pool rim with elbows braced against the wall, knees bent (Fig. 6-36). Now, using your elbows for leverage, swing your legs

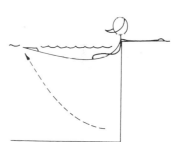

FIGURE 6-35

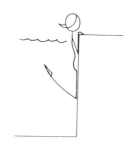

FIGURE 6-36

back until feet surface behind (Fig. 6-37). When this is easy, try it with knees straight. Finally, move arms into the basic SP and do the basic movement as suggested.

Two Choices. Do any version of **Nudibranch** with (1) ankles crossed or (2) soles of feet together, knees pressed sideward "frog" style.

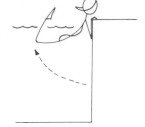

FIGURE 6-37

GOBY

Strengthens and stretches front/back of trunk

GET SET: In **water at least chin deep,** face the wall and hold the pool rim with hands shoulder-width apart, elbows braced against the wall. Dangle legs straight down, feet extended and together, stomach pulled in.

GO: Tip head forward as you tuck knees tightly to your chest (Fig. 6-38). Extend legs down to the SP, then press them back (Fig. 6-39). Move slowly from tuck to arch positions. As you tuck up, pull in your stomach hard, round your back, and exhale; as you arch, tighten buttocks, lift heels, tip head back, and inhale.

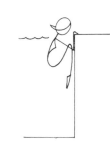

FIGURE 6-38

NOTE: While **Sea Whip, Nudibranch,** and **Goby** have similar arching movements, their starting and finishing positions are distinctly different.

HUMPBACK

A "whale" of an Aquacise to stretch the back, shoulders, chest, and to develop abdominal and pelvic control necessary for good posture

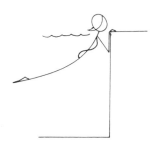

FIGURE 6-39

This and the next seven Aquacises (through **Pufferfish**) employ vigorous use of the Tuck-in and are especially helpful in developing pelvic control and, consequently, better posture.

GET SET: Face the wall in **waist-deep water** with your feet apart side to side. Bend forward from the hips and rest your hands on the ledge, shoulder-width apart.

GO: Lift your head and bend forward until you feel a stretch in shoulders and chest. Press your hips back as though someone were pulling you away from the wall (Fig. 6-40).

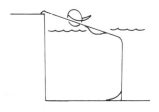

FIGURE 6-40

Next, pull in your stomach firmly, tip your head forward, and round your back (Fig. 6-41). Move slowly from one position to the other holding each for several seconds. Inhale as you arch; exhale as you Tuck-in. Start with 6 repetitions and work up to 12.

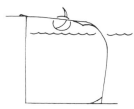

FIGURE 6-41

CLINGFISH

Strengthens abdomen and develops abdominal and pelvic control necessary for good posture. Variations also stretch chest area and strengthen upper back.

GET SET: Stand in **waist-to-chest-deep water** with your back against the wall, legs forward at an angle, feet braced against the floor (Fig. 6-42). Bend knees slightly and hold arms sideward, hands resting on the ledge, elbows straight.

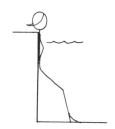

FIGURE 6-42

GO: Alternate between the following positions and repeat the sequence 6 times in the beginning. Gradually work up to 12. (1) Arch your lower back away from the wall, keeping buttocks, upper back, and arms in place (Fig. 6-43). (2) Tuck-in strongly to press the arch out of lower back and bring it against the wall. Inhale as you arch; exhale as you Tuck-in. If you like, hold the Tuck-in position as you inhale and exhale several times.

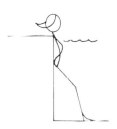

FIGURE 6-43

VARIATIONS:

Elbows Up. With lower back against the wall, hands clasped behind your head (which is held vigorously erect), squeeze shoulder blades together. Hold the contraction for several seconds. Relax and repeat three times. Avoid holding your breath.

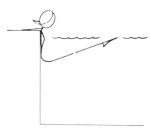

FIGURE 6-44

Fancy Clingfish (Shallow Water). Start again with back against the wall, arms sideward. However, this time brace your elbows on the pool ledge and extend legs forward, extended feet together and close to the surface. Tip your head forward, pull in your stomach hard, and stretch your legs (Fig. 6-44). Now, tip head back, arch your lower back, and bend your knees, touching feet to the wall (Fig. 6-45). Move slowly back to the SP, pulling in your stomach as you do. Contract and arch smoothly, holding each position for several seconds. Start with 6 repetitions and work up to 12.

Fancy Clingfish (Deep Water). Swimmers, suspend yourself in deep water with arms resting on the pool ledge. Bring legs forward, feet either together or apart. Now, perform these

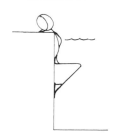

FIGURE 6-45

movements in sequence: (1) Pull in your stomach hard and flex your feet, pushing heels forward. (2) Extend your feet and press legs down until back and legs are against the wall. (As you do this, stretch legs and tighten buttocks). (3) Tip head back and arch your back. Fig. 6-46 (heels will slide several inches up the wall). (4) Pull in stomach hard, flatten back against the wall, and lift legs forward to the SP. Move smoothly from contracted to arched positions, holding each for several seconds. Start with 6 repetitions and work up to 12.

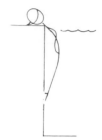

FIGURE 6-46

FLATFISH

Helps to flatten upper back for better posture

GET SET: Stand in **chest-deep water** with your back flat against the wall, legs forward at an angle, feet braced against the floor (Fig. 6-50). Hold arms down at your sides, the back of your hands and thumbs against the wall. Tuck-in tightly to bring lower back against the wall and hold head erect.

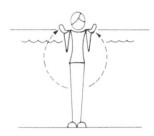

FIGURE 6-47

GO: Bend elbows and slowly slide thumbs up the wall toward your shoulders, keeping elbows close to your sides (Fig. 6-47). Reverse the motion and bring hands down to the start. Begin with 6 repetitions and work up to 10.

REMEMBER: (1) Keep your back, elbows, and thumbs against the wall throughout the movement. (2) Keep elbows close to your sides. Sounds easy—but it's not!

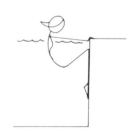

FIGURE 6-48

OYSTER

Develops abdominal and pelvic control for good posture; stretches back and firms abdomen

GET SET: Begin in the position shown in Fig. 6-48 with head tipped forward, back rounded, elbows straight. Pull in your stomach hard.

GO: Tip your head back and arch your back (Fig. 6-49). Move smoothly from one position to the other, holding each for a few seconds. Inhale as you arch; exhale as you contract.

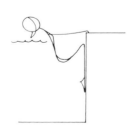

FIGURE 6-49

ARCHERFISH

Alternately Tuck-in and stretch to improve posture and release tension

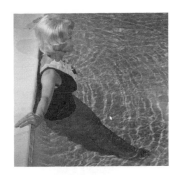

GET SET: Stand in **waist-to-chest-deep water** with your back toward the wall and hold onto the ledge with arms sideward, elbows straight.

GO: Each Aquacise in this group starts with a different position, but all combine the Tuck-in with cervical and lumbar hyper-extension. Do them gently, especially in the beginning. Start with 6 repetitions and gradually increase to 12.

FIGURE 6-50

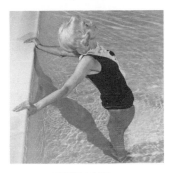

Touch Back—Chest Up. Stand with your back against the wall, legs forward, feet braced against the floor. Tuck-in to bring your lower back against the wall (Fig. 6-50). Now, do these movements in sequence: (1) Shove hips forward as you rise to the balls of your feet and slide hands closer together. (2) Inhale and arch (tip head back, lift chest, tighten buttocks, Fig. 6-51). (3) Exhale and return to the SP in one smooth motion, sliding hands along the ledge to bring your upper back, then your hips, to the wall. (4) Reaffirm your Tuck-in. Repeat several times, then try the movement keeping one leg forward, toes at the surface (Fig. 6-52). Stretch leg forward as if being pulled by the toes. After several repetitions, change to the other leg.

FIGURE 6-51

Sit Down—Stand Up. Stand in **lower-chest-deep water** and hold the rim securely. To start, bend your knees and brace the soles of your feet low on the wall, feet far apart (Fig. 6-53). Tuck-in. Repeat these movements in sequence: (1) Straighten your knees and lean forward arching your body, Fig. 6-54. (2) Hold briefly, then bend knees to the SP. (3) Reaffirm your Tuck-in and repeat. (4) After several repetitions, stretch your back by bringing upper back against the wall, then tuck up knees by lifting them above the surface (Fig. 6-55). Hold the stretch for several seconds before lowering feet to the SP. Inhale during (1) above, exhale during (2).

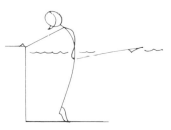

FIGURE 6-52

Chest Up—Backside Up. (Perform only in a smooth-sided pool.) This time, start with your feet together, heels close to the wall. Lean away from the wall and arch (Fig. 6-56). Now, do these movements in sequence: (1) Pull in your stomach and move hips back against the wall. (2) Immediately bend forward to a tight pike position (as head moves forward, backside will slide up the wall, Fig. 6-57). (3) Reverse the

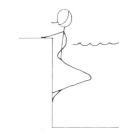

FIGURE 6-53

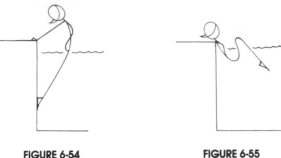

FIGURE 6-54 **FIGURE 6-55**

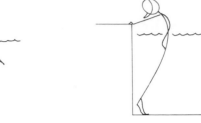

FIGURE 6-56

sequence and move smoothly back to the SP. Alternate from one position to the other holding each briefly. *Remember:* (1) Tip head forward to pike. (2) Pike tightly, pressing chest toward thighs. (3) Inhale as you arch. Begin to exhale as hips move back and continue to exhale until your face is again above the surface. Exhale through your nose or wear a nose clip and exhale through your mouth.

SPINY LOBSTER

Reinforces the Tuck-in habit; strengthens abdomen and buttocks

GET SET: In **waist-deep water,** brace your back against the wall with legs forward at an angle, feet braced against the pool floor, knees straight. Water should be at chest level when in position. Hold arms down at your sides against the wall, palms facing forward.

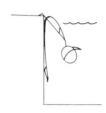

FIGURE 6-57

GO: Tuck-in strongly and press hips forward until body is straight, shoulders braced against the wall (Fig. 6-58). (Roll up one vertebra at a time, beginning at the base of your spine.) Reaffirm your Tuck-in and roll down to the start, bringing hips to the wall last. Inhale as hips move forward; exhale as they move back to the start. Repeat 6 times and gradually work up to 12.

STICKLEBACK

Reinforces Tuck-in habit for good body alignment; strengthens abdomen, upper body, and arms; increases flexibility of hip joints

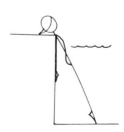

FIGURE 6-58

GET SET: With your back flat against the wall, brace your arms on the ledge. Bend knees and brace the soles of your feet on the wall, feet wide apart, heels close to buttocks. Tuck-in.

GO: Slowly press knees left toward the wall (Fig. 6-59). Move knees forward and Tuck-in to bring lower back against the wall. Repeat several times, alternating sides. Afterward, stretch your back by tucking knees up to your chest. Try to lift them above the surface (Fig. 6-55).

NOTE: To further strengthen abdominal muscles, add the following isometric contraction during the Tuck-in portion of the **Humpback, Oyster, Spiny Lobster,** and **Stickelback** movements: Pull in your stomach hard and hold for a slow count of eight. Relax and repeat twice more. Avoid holding your breath.

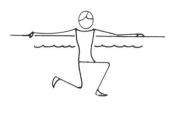

FIGURE 6-59

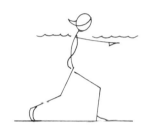

FIGURE 6-60

PUFFERFISH

Increases chest and shoulder flexibility; improves posture and relieves tension

Use **Pufferfish** to stretch and catch your breath after other, more vigorous Aquacises.

GET SET: Stand in **waist-to-chest-deep water** with feet far apart front to back. Bend knees to bring the **water level over your shoulders.** Hold arms forward at the surface and tip your head forward slightly (Fig. 6-60). Tuck-in.

GO: Lift your chest and inhale deeply while moving arms and head back (Fig. 6-61). Return arms and head to the forward SP while exhaling completely. (During this time, Tuck-in strongly.) Move hands along the surface of the water. Begin with only four repetitions and gradually increase to eight.

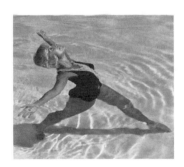

FIGURE 6-61

VARIATIONS:

Lift Leg and Return. Perform the basic movement but, as arms move forward, lift the forward leg high and touch fingers to toes (Fig. 6-62). Return leg to the start as arms move back.

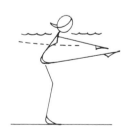

FIGURE 6-62

Periodically change leg position and perform with opposite leg.

Lift Leg and Hold. Perform the first variation with one leg forward the entire time. Move arms forward to bring fingers to toes, then move arms and head back as you press hips and leg forward. (Stretch leg as if being pulled forward by the toes, Fig. 6-63.) Repeat several times before performing with the opposite leg forward.

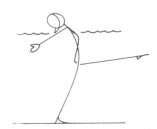

FIGURE 6-63

FEATHER DUSTER

Tones muscles of lower trunk and thighs; increases flexibility of spine and hip joints; develops posture awareness

GET SET: Hold a kickboard under each arm or use inflated swim wings for support, then move into **water at least chin deep.**[10] Hold each board out to the side with arms on top, fingers gripping the outer edges (Fig. 6-64). If using swim wings, hold one in each hand or wear one on each wrist with arms extended sideward in a wide V and relaxed. Larger wings may be slipped onto the upper arms for added support. Or, if using small ones, you may need two pairs—one in each hand and one on each wrist. Some people may find swim wings less stressful than kickboards to hands, arms, and shoulders.

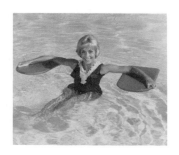

FIGURE 6-64

GO: Choose your favorites from this group, then do them VERY slowly while constantly stretching legs and body.

Pause 'n Stretch. Suspend yourself vertically, legs together. Tuck-in tightly, then stretch and tense your legs with feet extended, toes reaching toward the floor (Fig. 6-65). At the same time, lift your chest and stretch your body as much as possible. Breathe normally and hold the stretch for several seconds. Relax and repeat, this time with feet flexed and heels pressed toward the floor.

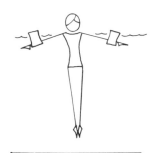

FIGURE 6-65

One Up. With body vertical and feet together, **Pause 'n Stretch** briefly. Then, keeping legs stretched, slowly lift one leg until toes touch hand (Fig. 6-66). Slowly press leg down and repeat with the other leg. Feet may be flexed or extended. To vary, lift leg across and touch toes to opposite hand.

Split to V—Pike—Press Down. With body vertical, feet together, **Pause 'n Stretch** briefly. Now, keeping legs stretched, slowly open them up to a high V-split, trying to bring toes to hands

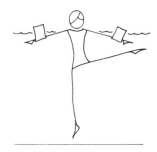

FIGURE 6-66

[10] Nonswimmers should not rely on floating devices for safety.

(Fig. 6-67). Next, move legs together in front to a pike position (Fig. 6-70) then slowly press them down to the start. Repeat several times, then do the reverse motion (first lift legs forward) or alternate one with the other.

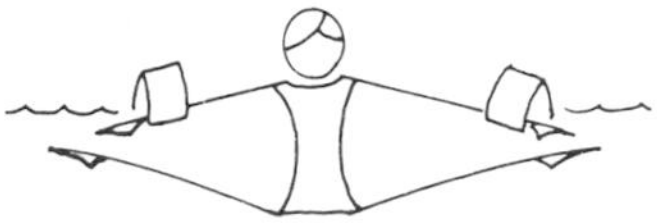

Swing Down and Cross. Begin with legs in a high V-split, toes at the surface. Press legs down to vertical and cross ankles. Then, lift legs forward to pike position (ankles still crossed). Reverse the action by pressing legs down to vertical, then separate them to the high V-split. During pike, lift legs as high as possible so that you are eventually able to bring them into the tight pike shown in Fig. 6-68. To vary, stop to **Pause 'n Stretch** each time legs move down to vertical.

Giant Steps. With body vertical, walk slowly forward through the water using giant steps. Lift one knee at a time toward your chest while flexing your foot (Fig. 6-69). Push heel far forward, straightening knee, then extend foot and press leg down to the start. Use smooth leg action, lift knees high, and reach feet foward as far as possible.

Twist 'n Step. Take **Giant Steps,** twisting at the waist and lifting each knee across to the opposite elbow. Lift knees high. You will stay in place during this Aquacise.

Hip Ahoy. Start with trunk erect, legs piked, toes at the surface (Fig. 6-70). Pull in your stomach hard. Now, inhale and shove your hips up to the surface as you tighten your buttocks (Fig. 6-71). Then, exhale and press hips down to the start. Keep legs stretched, feet extended, and toes at the surface. Also do this Aquacise with legs apart in a wide V; then, as hips move down, try to bring toes to hands (or boards).

Chug. Slowly inch your way forward through the water with this Aquacise, holding each tuck, pike, and vertical position briefly. Start with body vertical, legs together, then **Pause 'n Stretch.** Next, inhale and tuck up knees (Fig. 6-72). Straighten legs

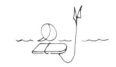

FIGURE 6-67

FIGURE 6-68

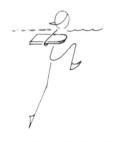

FIGURE 6-69

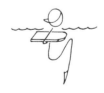

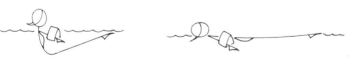

FIGURE 6-70

FIGURE 6-71

FIGURE 6-72

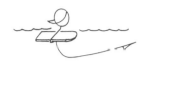

FIGURE 6-73

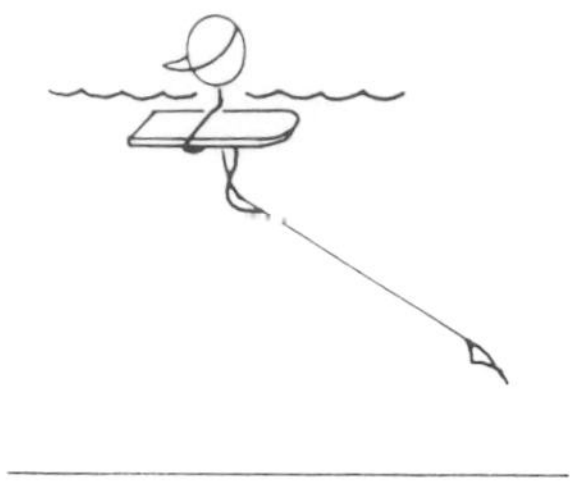

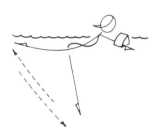

FIGURE 6-74

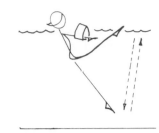

FIGURE 6-75

forward (Fig. 6-73) then exhale as you thrust hips forward and press legs down to the start (Fig. 6-74). Remember to tighten buttocks when pushing hips forward and always keep trunk erect. Lifting legs too high will cause you to lean back too far to use legs effectively.

Scissors. Start with body vertical, legs stretched, and feet extended, then **Pause 'n Stretch.** Next, slowly swing legs back and forth scissors fashion. Perform some scissors with trunk slanted back to bring toes to the surface in front (Fig. 6-75) and some with trunk slanted forward to bring heels to the surface in back (Fig. 6-76). Separate legs as far as possible during scissors.

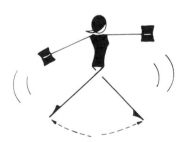

FIGURE 6-76

Swivel. Stretch out front-down on the surface of the water, with arms sideward and head up. Start with legs stretched and separated in a wide V-split, feet extended (Fig. 6-77). Now, twist at the waist, turning hips to the right as you slowly press right leg back, left leg forward into a scissors-split position (upper leg at the surface Fig. 6-78). Turn hips forward again as you slowly move legs together to the SP. Repeat to the left, moving the left leg back and right leg forward. Move smoothly from V- to scissors-split positions holding each while stretching legs far apart. (If you concentrate on pressing the upper leg back, your hips will turn automatically.)

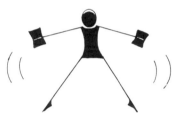

FIGURE 6-77

Tuck—Tip. Start on your back, knees tucked high to chest (Fig. 6-79). Now, keeping knees bent, straighten at the hip joint and press knees down and up to the back until feet emerge above the surface (Figs. 6-80 and 6-81). Reverse the motion, tucking knees up and tipping back to the start.

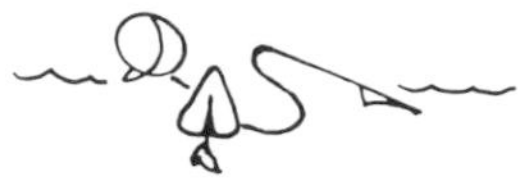

FIGURE 6-78

Pike—Arch. Move your legs slowly from pike to arch, holding each position briefly. Start with body vertical, legs together. **Pause 'n Stretch.** Now, with trunk upright, pike legs to bring toes to the surface (Fig. 6-82). Next, press legs down and back,

FIGURE 6-79

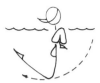

FIGURE 6-80

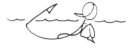

FIGURE 6-81

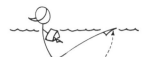

FIGURE 6-82

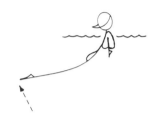

FIGURE 6-83

tightening buttocks and lifting chest (Fig. 6-83). Reverse the motion, pressing legs down past the SP and up to the front. Inhale as legs move up; exhale as they move down. Try this also with ankles crossed. And, if you like, move arms forward as legs move forward; move them back as legs move back.

Tuck—Tip—Extend. Start on your back with legs straight and together. Tuck knees to chest, then tip forward to your stomach and straighten legs onto the surface in back. Reverse the motion tucking knees up and tipping back to the SP. Also try this with ankles crossed.

Split—Tip. Start on your back, legs together, toes at the surface. Now, sit down in the water as you separate legs to a wide V-split. Continue to press legs apart and around to the back as you tip forward to your stomach. Bring legs together in back (Figs. 6-84, 6-85, and 6-86). Next, reverse the motion, separating legs to a wide V and lowering hips again as legs move forward. Keep legs far apart as you tip over.

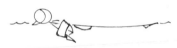

FIGURE 6-84

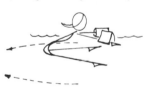

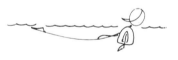

FIGURE 6-86

FIGURE 6-85

Frog Knees to High V-Split

1. Start with body vertical, feet together. **Pause 'n Stretch.** Now, slowly bend your knees and lift them to your elbows while flexing feet (Fig. 6-87). Next, try to keep knees at the same elevation as you straighten them to a high V-split and touch toes to fingers. (With swim wings, you can grasp your toes and hold the stretch for several seconds, Fig. 6-88.) Slowly press legs down to the start while extending feet.

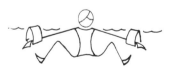

FIGURE 6-87

2. Perform **Frog Knees** to the high V-split, then move legs forward and pike before extending feet and pressing legs down to the start.

3. Perform **Frog Knees** to the high V-split, then swing legs together in back as you tip forward to your stomach. Press legs down as you move trunk to the vertical SP.

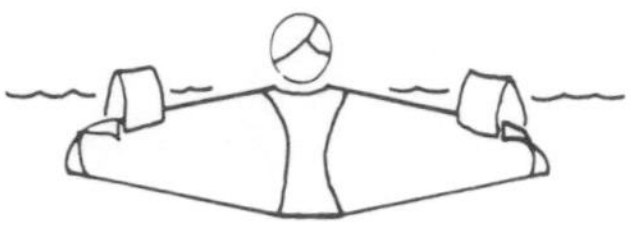

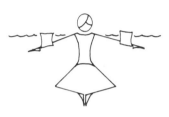

Frog Knees 'n Swing

1. Start with body vertical. Press knees outward and put the soles of your feet together (Fig. 6-89). Now, swing your knees pendulum style, first up to one side (Fig. 6-90), then down past the start and up to the other side. Keep knees pressed apart as you try to lift them up to your hands.

2. Start with body vertical. Press knees outward with soles of feet together. Now, keeping feet together, knees apart, swing legs forward and back. Lift feet to the surface in front (tip over to your back), then swing feet down and up to the surface in back (tip forward to your front).

FIGURE 6-88

Arc Side to Side. Start with body vertical, legs straight and together. **Pause 'n Stretch.** Hold the stretch as you swing legs from side to side, pendulum style, feet either extended or flexed. Try to bring side of body and legs close to the surface (Fig. 6-91). It's easier if you inhale and stretch the lower arm as legs rise; exhale as they descend. For a change, hold the side position for a slow count of eight while stretching to your limit with buttocks, stomach, and leg muscles taut.

FIGURE 6-89

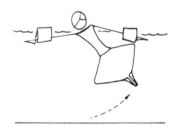

Tuck—Extend Side. Start with trunk vertical, knees tucked up to chest. Keeping legs together, tip onto one side and straighten legs sideward to the position shown in Fig. 6-91. Tuck knees again, then reverse the motion to the other side.

FIGURE 6-90

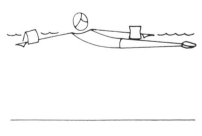

FIGURE 6-91

REMEMBER: When doing **Feather Duster** Aquacises: (1) Move extra slowly. (2) Constantly stretch/tense your legs and extend your feet strongly. (3) Pull in your stomach. (4) Lift toes to the surface during pike; lift knees to the surface during tuck. (5) Tighten buttocks as you press legs down or back. (6) Inhale as legs move up; exhale as legs move down.

Among other movements that can be done with floating supports, see **Goby** (p. 110); and **Pipefish, Jollytail, Sand Bug, Scud,** and **Dragonfly** Aquacises from the "Trunk Shape-Ups" chapter.

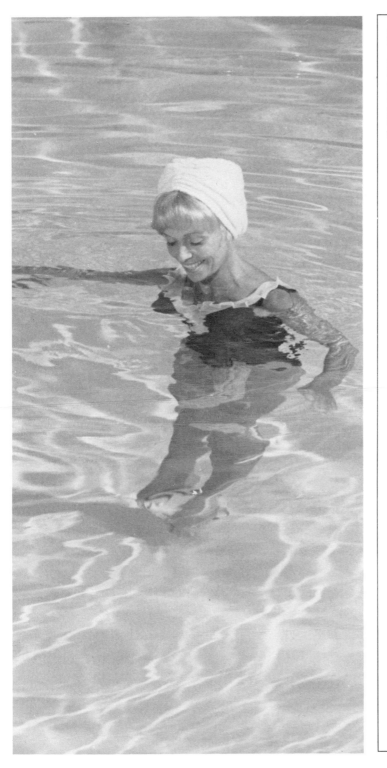

Part III
PADDLES, BOARDS, BALLS, AND WINGS

Part IV
PADDLES

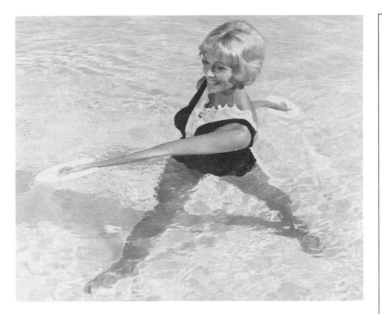

Chapter 7
PADDLE
AQUACISES

Paddle Aquacises, which I first introduced in 1973, have become an integral part of the Aquacises system of exercise. The notion of using paddles for extra resistance is my interpretation of the principle used by many aquatic birds. Some use their wings to actually fly under the water; others dive into the water then turn and surface using their wings as oars.

Paddles provide more support than the hands alone during slow movements and add greater resistance during faster movements. Most Paddle Aquacises are done in the shallow water with the face above the surface and only a few require basic swimming skills. Paddle Aquacises (1) strengthen and firm muscles of the hands, arms, shoulders, chest, and back, (2) increase flexibility in shoulders and chest, (3) improve posture, and (4) firm and trim the waist and stomach, or hips and thighs (as in **Paddlefish, Thresher,** etc.). In addition to contributing to overall fitness, Paddle Aquacises help to improve basic swimming skills so that you are more at ease in the water. For beginning swimmers, they help to coordinate breathing with the front crawl arm stroke (often a seemingly impossible feat) by stabilizing the body when turning the head to inhale. Moreover, paddles provide extra power to slide quickly through the water when stroking and sculling.

Paddle Aquacises

PADDLEFISH (p. 127)
  Dip Down and Up
  Ripple the Surface
  Add a Twist
  Dip Down—Cross and Lift
GRIBBLE (p. 128)
  Basic Movement
MUSKRAT (p. 128)
  Basic Movement
WATER STRIDER (p. 129)
  Basic Movement
THRESHER (p. 129)
  Basic Movement
PIRANHA (p. 129)
  Basic Movement
SEA ROBIN (p. 130)
  Basic Movement
  Fancy Sea Robin
SAILFISH (p. 130)
  Basic Movement
  Super Sailfish

PLATYPUS (p. 131)
  Basic Movement
  Press 'n Clap
SKIMMER (p. 131)
  Basic Movement
SCALLOP (p. 132)
  Basic Movement
  Upward Arm Recovery
CRAB (p. 132)
  Sit Down—Reach Out
  Stand Up—Reach Out
  Reach out and Twist
  Out 'n In
HUMUHUMU (p. 133)
  Knees Up and Swing
  Legs Up and Swing
  V-Split—Swing and Touch
RAY (p. 134)
  One Knee Up—Clap
  Both Knees Up—Clap
  Kick—Clap Sequence
  Follow Through—Clap
  V-Split—Clap

PADDLE POINTERS

1. Grip paddles with fingers curved through the slots, thumbs hooked underneath, or with fingers straight on the top surface. (Use this grip also for swim strokes.) To order paddles, see information at the back of this book.
2. All Paddle Aquacises are done with the hands below the surface.
3. The water level is essential to the effectiveness of most Paddle Aquacises and is noted in each instruction. If the water is too shallow, it makes it difficult to keep your hands beneath the surface and to perform the movement correctly. Conversely, water that is too deep hampers body stability and, therefore, minimizes resistance to your movements.
4. Move slowly in the beginning until strength and flexibility improve; then, increase the range and speed of your movements and gradually increase the number of times you repeat each Aquacise.

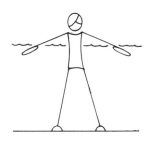

FIGURE 7-1

PADDLEFISH

Firms muscles of the trunk and arms; increases flexibility of chest and shoulders

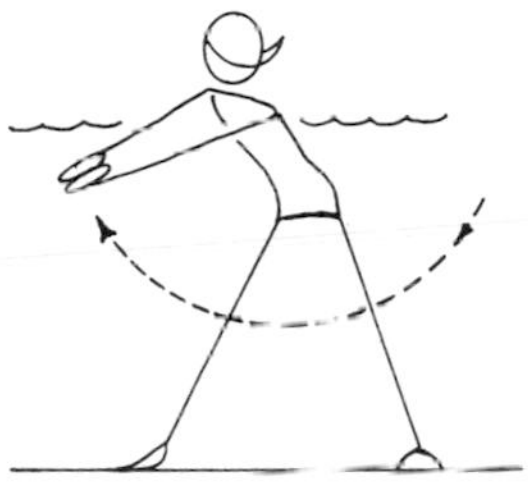

GET SET: Hold a paddle in each hand and stand in **chest-deep water** with feet apart side to side. Extend arms sideward and back, hands at the surface, palms down (Fig. 7-1).

GO: Choose your favorites from this group and repeat each 6 to 12 times to each side. Keep elbows straight, heels on the floor, and stomach pulled in.

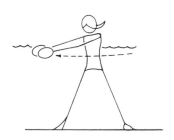

FIGURE 7-2

Dip Down and Up. Swing one arm down past your legs and up to meet the other hand (Fig. 7-2). Reverse the motion to the SP and repeat, alternating arms. For a change, perform in waist-deep water with your trunk bent forward from the hips. Keep back straight.

Ripple the Surface. Start in the **Get Set** position but with palms facing forward. Swing one arm across to meet the other hand, keeping paddle just under the surface (Fig. 7-3). Reverse the motion back to the SP and repeat, alternating arms.

Add a Twist. Start in the **Get Set** position (but with palms facing forward) then twist to the right. Next, swing the left arm across

FIGURE 7-3

to meet the right, then swing left arm back to the side as you turn to face front. Immediately twist left, then swing right arm across to the left. During the twist, stretch arms back as if an imaginary pole were extended across your shoulders from fingertip to fingertip.

Dip Down — Cross and Lift. Press arms straight down and across your body, moving one arm across in front, the other across in back. Continue the motion by twisting at the waist and lifting the paddles up to the surface, palms up (Fig. 7-4). Reverse the motion by pressing arms down, turn to face front, and lift arms sideward. Keep hands in a fixed position. Perform in a like manner, twisting to the other side.

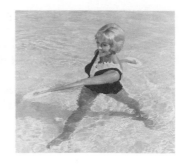

FIGURE 7-4

GRIBBLE

Strengthens wrists and forearms

GET SET: Stand in **chest-deep water,** feet apart side to side. Hold a paddle in each hand, and extend arms forward, shoulder-width apart. Hold paddles just under the surface, palms facing one another.

GO: Alternately bend hands back at the wrists, then forward, touching tips of paddles together. Keep arm motion to a minimum by confining the action to your hands. Repeat 6 to 12 times. Next, perform with arms sideward, palms turned to face front. Finally, perform with arms down in a low V. Swing hands up and down, touching tips of paddles to legs on the downward motion (Fig. 7-5).

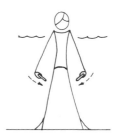

FIGURE 7-5

MUSKRAT

A total-body exercise for swimmers

GET SET: Hold a paddle in each hand and stretch out, front down, on the surface of the water. Hold your head up, arms forward.

GO: Flutter kick as you move the paddles apart then toward each other in a vigorous sculling motion, skimming them through the surface. Try to "swim" in place (Fig. 7-6) until pleasantly tired. Rest briefly, then repeat. For the arm motion, swing arms outward, tilting paddles to angle thumbs down slightly; swing arms inward, angling thumbs up. If coordination is difficult at first, practice the arm movement while standing; then lie front down and add the leg motion.

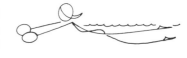

FIGURE 7-6

WATER STRIDER

Great for all-over toning and stretching for swimmers and floaters

GET SET: Ease into a back floating position with a paddle in each hand, arms at your sides with palms facing legs.

GO: Open arms and legs sideward to the position shown in Fig. 7-7, then close them forcefully to the SP. Keep hands under the surface. **Water Strider** will move you head first across the pool.

REMEMBER: (1) Stretch from head to toes, with head in line with body (look skyward). (2) Tuck-in. (3) Keep elbows and knees straight, feet extended.

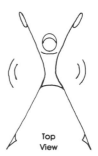

FIGURE 7-7

THRESHER

Fine for all-over stretching and firming

GET SET: Stand in **waist-to-chest-deep water** with your right side facing the wall. Hold the ledge with your right hand, a paddle in your left hand. Raise left arm and leg to the side. Turn palm to face front with paddle just under the surface.

GO: Swing left arm and leg forward and back horizontally in opposition to one another. (Swing arm back as you swing leg forward, Fig. 7-8; swing leg back, arm forward, Fig. 7-9). Lean forward and stretch when arm is forward; lean back when arm is back. Also do this Aquacise with right leg and arm, left side toward the wall. Start with 8 and work up to 20 repetitions for each side. If coordination is difficult at first, practice leg and arm motions separately.

REMEMBER: (1) Swing leg through a wide arc, keeping foot extended and close to the surface, knee straight. (2) Keep hand in a fixed position for greatest water resistance.

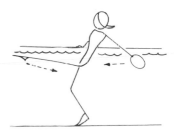

FIGURE 7-8

PIRANHA

Increases shoulder flexibility and firms arms and shoulders

GET SET: Stand with feet apart side to side in **shoulder-deep water.** Hold arms sideward and back as far as possible, palms facing up.

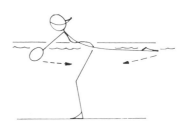

FIGURE 7-9

GO: Rapidly rotate your arms to turn palms alternately down and up. Next, repeat with arms forward, then with arms down at your sides. Rotate 6 to 12 times with arms in each position, and repeat the sequence one or more times.

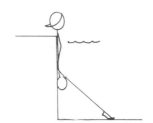

SEA ROBIN

Strengthens and firms upper body, shoulders, and arms; increases shoulder joint flexibility

FIGURE 7-10

GET SET: Stand in **chest-deep water** with your back flat against the wall, legs forward at an angle, feet on floor. Hold a paddle in each hand with arms at your sides (Fig. 7-10). Rotate arms outward, turning palms to face away from body (elbows face toward body). Tuck-in.

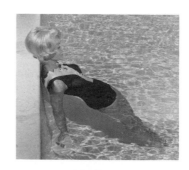

GO: Keeping the edge of paddles close to the wall, lift arms sideward to the surface, then turn palms down and press arms down. Turn palms to face out again and repeat the up-down motion 5 to 10 times. Next, do **Sea Robin** starting with arms rotated inward. (Palms face away from body again, but this time elbows face outward.) Keep back against the wall by Tucking-in.

FIGURE 7-11

VARIATION:

Fancy Sea Robin. Perform both of the above movements from the position shown in Fig. 7-11 with the water at shoulder level. Rest your shoulders and neck against the wall and brace your toes against the floor. Tuck-in tightly to keep body straight and stiff.

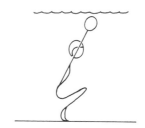

FIGURE 7-12

SAILFISH

An excellent body conditioner for swimmers

GET SET: Stand in **shoulder-deep water,** a paddle in each hand, arms at your sides.

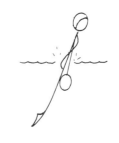

GO: Scoop arms up to lower yourself into a squatting position beneath the surface (Fig. 7-12). Now, forcefully pull your arms down and push your feet off pool floor, thrusting yourself upward and stretching from head to extended feet (Fig. 7-13). At the height of the jump, scoop arms up to descend to the squatting position. Inhale through your mouth when face is above the surface; exhale through mouth and nose when under the water. Repeat 10 times and gradually increase to 20.

FIGURE 7-13

VARIATION:

Super Sailfish. Try **Sailfish** in deeper water. See how high you can lift yourself and how deep you can descend on each up-down arm motion. Just remember that the paddles give you extra momentum and you will "fly" to the bottom faster than if you used hands alone. For greater challenge, do **Super Sailfish** to move across the deep end of the pool.

PLATYPUS

Stretches back of legs; firms arms and trunk

GET SET: In **chest-deep water,** stand with your back against the wall, legs forward at an angle, feet braced against the floor. Hold arms sideward against the wall, hands just under the surface, palms facing forward. Lift your right leg forward, toes at the surface, knee straight. Pull in your stomach.

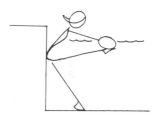

FIGURE 7-14

GO: Keeping hips against the wall, sweep arms forward and touch paddles to toes (Fig. 7-14) then sweep arms back to the start. Next, turn palms down and press arms down to your sides. Lift arms up to the start; turn palms to face front and repeat the entire movement 4 to 12 times before changing to the left leg. Keep leg high, hands under the surface.

VARIATION:

Press 'n Clap. As arms move down, press hips forward, then clap hands behind hips (Fig. 7-15); lift arms to the side as you move hips back to the wall.

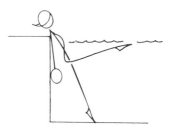

SKIMMER

Strengthens and firms muscles of arms and trunk, especially the waist

FIGURE 7-15

GET SET: Stand in **waist-to-chest-deep water** with feet apart side to side. Hold a paddle in each hand, arms forward at the surface, shoulder-width apart, palms down.

GO: Skim paddles through the surface as you twist from side to side. Press down on the paddles as you tilt palms slightly in the direction of motion. Keep heels on the pool floor, stomach pulled in. Start with 10 repetitions and gradually increase to 20.

SCALLOP

Firms arms, chest, and abdomen

GET SET: Stand in **chest-deep water** with your feet together, then bend your knees to bring the water level to your shoulders. Extend arms sideward and back as far as possible, hands just under the surface, palms slanted forward (Fig. 7-16).

GO: Jet propel yourself backward across the shallow end of the pool. To do this, use the **Reverse Oarfish** arm motion (p. 27) and simultaneously scoop arms forward and lift your feet (Fig. 7-17). Glide backward briefly, then bend knees and elbows and return feet to the floor, arms to the sideward SP. For maximum backward momentum, jump up lightly, thrusting your hips back as you vigorously scoop arms forward. During the glide, pull in your stomach even more, lift your legs high, and reach toward your toes. Start with 10 and work up to 20 repititions.

VARIATION:

Upward Arm Recovery. For extra stretch to the shoulders, use an above-the-surface arm recovery. To do this, scoop arms forward and lift feet as instructed. Then, as you lower feet to the floor, swing arms overhead and down to the side SP. Have paddles enter the water in preparation for the next forward scoop when arms are sideward and back as far as possible.

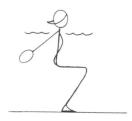

FIGURE 7-16

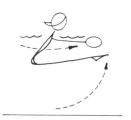

FIGURE 7-17

CRAB

Improves posture; firms arms, shoulders, and trunk. **The last two versions incorporate a twist and thus add waist exercise.**

GET SET: Use the starting positions given for each of the following Aquacises.

GO: Repeat any of your favorites 8 times in the beginning and gradually work up to 20. Swing paddles just under the surface so they ripple the water.

Sit Down—Reach Out. Stand with your back against the wall in **waist-deep water;** then, bend your knees to bring the water to chest level. Hold the paddles against your midsection with elbows sideward against the wall. Tuck-in. Now, open arms sideward until elbows are straight, the back of your hands touching the wall. Reverse the motion pulling hands forward to the SP. Keep elbows and back flat against the wall the entire time so that all the action occurs in the lower arm.

Stand Up—Reach Out. Stand away from the wall in **chest-deep water** with feet apart side to side, paddles against your midsection (Fig. 7-18). Now, perform the arm movement described above. For variation, do it with one arm at a time, using arms alternately.

Reach Out and Twist. Perform **Stand Up—Reach Out** and add a twist at the waist as you open arms sideward (Fig. 7-19). Then turn forward as you pull hands back to the start. Twist to alternate sides. For variation, perform with one arm at a time (i.e., press right arm sideward as you twist right; pull hand to midsection as you turn to face front. Repeat with the left arm and twist to the left).

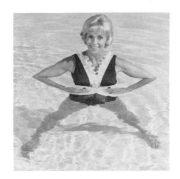

FIGURE 7-18

Out 'n In. Standing in **chest-deep water** with feet either together or apart to the side, perform **Crab** by moving arms in opposition to one another. In other words, press one arm sideward as you pull the other hand to your midsection. If you bend your knees and balance on the balls of your feet, the arm movement will cause your hips to rotate from side to side.

HUMUHUMU

Excellent conditioner for the arms and trunk, especially the waist and abdomen. For swimmers only.

GET SET: Stand in **chin-deep water** and extend arms forward in a wide V at the surface, a paddle in each hand.

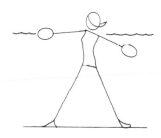

FIGURE 7-19

GO: Start with the first and easiest movement before trying the other more difficult ones. The side to side arm and leg motions are the same for each version—only the leg position varies. Keep your stomach pulled in and repeat each movement until arm or stomach muscles become fatigued. If coordination of arms and legs is difficult at first, practice the arm movement alone while standing.

Knees Up and Swing. Tuck up knees, then swing arms and knees from side to side, moving arms in the opposite direction of your knees. (Swing knees toward left elbow as arms swing right, then toward right elbow as arms swing left.) Feel the twisting action in your waist as you swing knees far to each side. Swing continuously, keeping hands just under the surface and palms tilted in the direction of motion. Keep legs together and tucked up high.

Legs Up and Swing. Perform the above movement, but with legs straight and together, feet extended and close to the surface. Touch opposite hand to foot (Fig. 7-20). Even better, strive to swing legs far to the side, moving them past hands.

V-Split—Swing and Touch. This time, perform **Humuhumu** with legs apart in a high, wide V-split, toes close to the surface. As you swing arms and legs in opposition to one another, reach across touching hand to opposite foot. Keep legs stretched and feet extended.

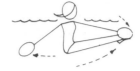

FIGURE 7-20

RAY

Firms muscles of the arms and trunk; the last three versions also firm hips and thighs

GET SET: Stand with feet together in **chest-deep water** holding the paddles with arms sideward, palms down (Fig. 7-21).

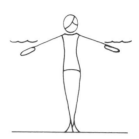

FIGURE 7-21

GO: Use these Aquacises separately by repeating the movement 6 to 20 times. Or, use several in a sequence by repeating each two to six times before moving to the next. The down-up lateral arm motion is the same in each version. Keep elbows and back straight, stomach pulled in.

One Knee Up—Clap. Simultaneously lift one knee toward your chest and press arms down clapping hands under thigh (Fig. 7-22). Reverse the action, returning to the SP and repeat, alternating legs.

Both Knees Up—Clap. Simultaneously tuck up both knees to your chest and clap hands under your thighs (Fig. 7-23). Reverse the motion to the SP. Keep legs together and lift knees high.

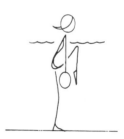

FIGURE 7-22

Kick—Clap Sequence. Kick one leg forward as you press arms down and clap hands under thigh (Fig. 7-24). Reverse the motion to the SP. Repeat several times, alternating legs. Next, do several more repetitions, this time kicking up to the back as you clap hands down in front (Fig. 7-25). Finally, repeat the action by kicking sideward (knee cap facing up, Fig. 7-26) and clapping down in front. Always keep knee of kicking leg straight and try to kick up to the surface; then press leg all the way down to the feet-together SP.

Follow Through—Clap. Kick forward with knee straight and clap under your thigh. However, this time swing leg down past

FIGURE 7-23

the start and up to the back as arms move up. Next, swing leg down and up to the front again as you press arms down and clap under thigh. Repeat several times before performing with the other leg.

V-Split—Clap. Start by standing on your toes with feet apart side to side. Now, simultaneously lift both legs sideward in a V-split as you press arms down to clap hands (Fig. 7-27). Reverse the motion back to the start.

NOTE: Avoid jumping up at the start of **Both Knees Up** and **V-Split.** Smooth pressure on the paddles is all you need to keep your head above the surface.

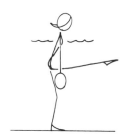

FIGURE 7-24

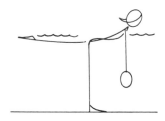

FIGURE 7-25

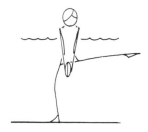

FIGURE 7-26

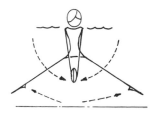

FIGURE 7-27

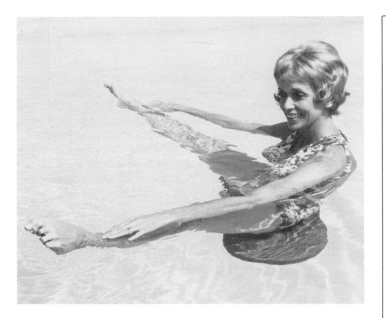

Kickboarding

"Kickboarding"—using swimming kicks while holding a kick-board—effectively improves your kicking skills, increases calorie consumption, and firms legs, hips, buttocks, and abdomen. In fact, it's an even more concentrated leg exercise than swimming because the legs do all the work. Kicking is also an excellent substitute for land jogging because it enables you to improve your cardiovascular fitness with much less stress to your joints. At the same time, kickboarding keeps your head out of the water so you can breathe more easily, see where you're going, and keep your hair dry. Clearly, the superb benefits derived from this slimming activity make it a valuable addition to your aquatic fitness program.

Basic swimming kicks or kicking variations can be used as follows:

1. As a warm-up before your Aquacise session.
2. Between Shape-Ups or other Aquacises in your session as a change of pace.
3. At the end of your session as an aid in developing greater muscle tone and cardiovascular fitness.

To make your kicks smoother and more beneficial, start with a brushup using the **Water Boatman** as a guide to basic kicking techniques. This will help prepare you for the more difficult kicking variations in **Surfbird.** For further variety, see

Kickboarding

WATER BOATMAN (Basic Kicking
Techniques) (p. 139)
    Flutter Kick on Your Front
    Flutter Kick on Your Back
    Breast Stroke Kick
    Elementary Backstroke Kick
    Sidestroke Kick

SURFBIRD (Kicking Variations) (p. 144)
    Flutter Kick Variations on your Front
    Flutter Kick Variations on Your Back
    Breast Stroke Kick Variations
    Elementary Backstroke Kick Variations
    Sidestroke Kick Variations

"More Kickboard Kapers." You will need a styrofoam kickboard (about 12 × 22 × 1½ inches) which can be purchased at many drug, pool supply, and sporting goods stores at very little cost. However, don't confuse them with styrofoam surfboards which are larger and unwieldy.

WATER BOATMAN

Basic Kicking Techniques

If you can swim, even a little, you can learn kickboarding. If not, substitute the "Walk, Jog, Jump, Hop, and Kick" (at the wall) chapter.

Making headway through the water using only the legs is sometimes difficult, even for fairly good swimmers who have relied on a strong arm stroke to compensate for a weak kick. If you have this problem, review your kick using the pointers below to help identify your trouble spot. If you need more help, find a competent Red Cross Water Safety instructor to get you on the right track. The kicking highlights in this section are intended to help you make the most of **Surfbird** kicking variations, but they will not substitute for lessons. If you are a beginning swimmer, stay in the shallow water and do your kicking across widths of the pool. DO NOT RELY ON THE KICKBOARD FOR SAFETY. First off, it's important to hold the board correctly to make smooth progress through the water, so . . .

GET SET TO FLUTTER KICK ON YOUR FRONT: Extend your arms forward and hold the board along the sides. Keep elbows straight and rest the board on the surface (Fig. 8-1). Breathe either by (1) lifting your face forward to inhale, then exhaling face down or (2) keeping your head up with your chin at water level. With your head up, your kick will be slightly deeper.

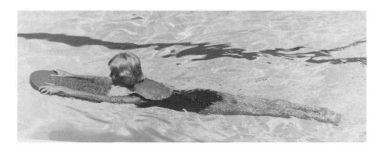

FIGURE 8-1

GO: To flutter kick on your front:

1. Swing your legs from the hips and relax your knees and ankles.
2. On the downward kick of each leg, drop your knee toward the pool floor, feeling the pressure of the water against your instep.
3. When your knee is straight, you have completed the downward phase of the kick.
4. On the upward phase, push up against the water with the soles of your feet and let your heels just break the surface.
5. Kick with ankles relaxed so that the resistance of the water forces your feet into an extended position. This helps to maintain headfirst progress.
6. Limit the depth of your kick to 12 to 18 inches and maintain a steady, even rhythm.
7. Students are sometimes unable to progress forward. Most often this is caused by (a) holding the feet in a rigid, flexed position, (b) kicking with stiff knees, or (c) over-bending the knee and kicking with only the lower leg. Once you spot your error, the secret is to go slowly until a new kicking pattern is established. There will be plenty of time later to add speed. These suggestions also apply to flutter kicking on your back.

GET SET TO FLUTTER KICK ON YOUR BACK: Hold the board with arms overhead, board resting on the surface, elbows straight (Fig. 8-2). However, to flutter kick, tuck chin slightly so that water line is along jaw and crown of head.

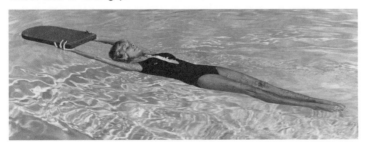

FIGURE 8-2

GO: To flutter kick on your back:

1. Swing your legs from the hips and relax your knees and ankles.
2. On the downward kick, drop your heel toward the pool floor, feeling the pressure of the water against the sole of your foot.

3. On the upward motion, kick as if kicking a football and feel the pressure of the water against your instep. Allow toes to just break the surface.

4. Your leg will be straight at the top of each kick, but keep your knees from breaking the surface.

5. Kick with ankles relaxed so that the resistance of the water forces your feet into an extended position. This helps maintain headfirst progress.

6. When flutter kicking on your back, most of the bending occurs at the knee rather than at the hip, so avoid a sitting position in the water.

7. Proper head position (tucking chin so that water line is along jaw and crown of head) helps prevent knees from breaking the surface.

8. Limit the depth of your kick to 15 to 18 inches and maintain a steady, even rhythm.

NOTE: For more resistance and to develop a correct and relaxed flutter kick pattern, try using swim fins during a portion of your practice.

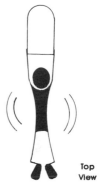

Top View

FIGURE 8-3

GET SET TO BREAST STROKE KICK: Hold the board as shown in Fig. 8-1.

GO: To breast stroke kick:

1. Start in a glide position (see #4 below).
2. On the first phase of the kick, perform the following movements *smoothly and simultaneously:*
   a. Drop your knees toward pool floor, knees separated a comfortable distance.
   b. Lift your heels toward your buttocks (heels 2 to 3 inches apart). Lift heels gently so that headfirst momentum is not disrupted.
   c. Flex your feet and bend your knees so that the soles of your feet are just under the surface and facing up (Fig. 8-3).
3. From this position, and in *one continuous motion,* turn your feet (feet still flexed) so that your toes point sideward and press your feet backward to the glide position (Fig. 8-4).
4. As you glide, stretch your legs and press them together, with feet extended. Hold the glide until you lose momentum.

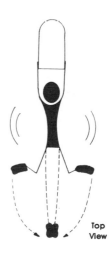

Top View

FIGURE 8-4

GET SET TO ELEMENTARY BACKSTROKE KICK: Lie on your back and hold the board as shown in Fig. 8-2.

GO: To kick elementary backstroke style (sometimes referred to as inverted breast stroke kick):

1. Start in a glide position (see #4 below).
2. On the first phase of the kick, perform the following movements *smoothly and simultaneously:*
   a. Bend your knees (90^n), dropping your heels toward the pool floor. Lower heels gently so that headfirst momentum is not disrupted.
   b. Separate your knees a comfortable distance.
   c. Flex your feet with heels 2 to 3 inches apart (Fig. 8-5).
3. From this position, and in *one continuous motion,* turn feet so that toes point sideward (feet still flexed) and press them outward and around to the glide position (Fig. 8-6). Press firmly to feel the resistance of the water on the inner edges of your feet.
4. As you glide, Tuck-in, stretch your legs, and press them together with feet extended. Body should be straight and close to the surface, head resting on the water. Look straight up. Hold the glide until you lose momentum.
5. Avoid sitting down in the water during the first phase of the kick. Bend mainly from the knee rather than at the hip to keep knees from breaking the surface.

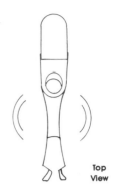

FIGURE 8-5

GET SET TO SIDESTROKE KICK: Either (1) lie on your right side as shown in Fig. 8-7. Hold the lower left corner of the board with your left hand and rest your right arm on top, fingers gripping the upper end of the board. Or (2) lie on one side holding the center bottom edge of the board with your lower hand and resting your upper arm on your side (Fig. 8-8). However, if you are more comfortable on your other side, use the opposite arm positions.

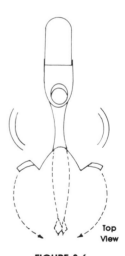

FIGURE 8-6

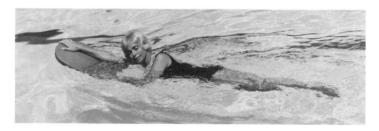

FIGURE 8-7

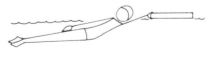

FIGURE 8-8

GO: To Sidestroke kick:

1. Start in a glide position (see #5 below).
2. Bend your knees up, keeping heels together and on a line with your buttocks (Fig. 8-9). At the same time, flex your feet and separate your knees 3 to 4 inches. Avoid crouching in the water by bending knees only a comfortable distance.
3. Separate your legs by moving the upper leg forward and the lower leg back (Fig. 8-10). Be sure to move the lower leg back as far as possible.
4. Without pausing, straighten your legs to a scissors-split position (Fig. 8-11) and press them together to glide. Avoid letting feet drift past one another.
5. As you glide, Tuck-in and stretch your legs with feet together and extended. Keep head in line with body, lower ear in the water, and hold the glide until you lose momentum.

NOTE: Advanced swimmers, for a change try your basic kicks without a board. For front kicks, stretch your arms forward, with your fingertips at the surface and head up. For side kicks, hold your top arm in a vertical position. For back kicks, stretch your arms overhead on the surface of the water, palms up, with one hand resting on the other. For a more difficult version of the back kick, hold your arms in a vertical position, with your fingers pointing toward the ceiling (Fig. 8-12).

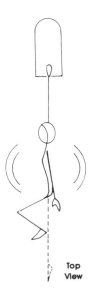

FIGURE 8-9

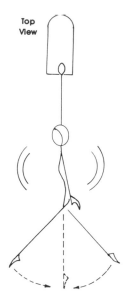

FIGURE 8-11

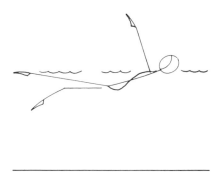

FIGURE 8-12

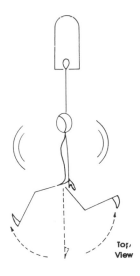

FIGURE 8-10

SURFBIRD

Kicking variations to develop endurance, and strenghten muscles of legs and lower trunk

GET SET: Hold the board as required for the following kicks. See explanations and illustrations for basic kicks in **Water Boatman.**

GO: Kick back and forth across lengths or widths of the pool using as many of these kicking styles as you like; however, do at least one length or width per style.

Flutter Kick Variations on Your Front

1. Kick slow, with legs deep in the water, head up.
2. Use short, fast kicks with feet close to the surface.
3. Kick slow to medium to fast, using eight kicks at each speed.
4. Alternate eight flutter kicks with four breast stroke kicks. Bring legs together before moving into breast stroke kick.
5. Alternate 16 flutter kicks with 2 sidestroke kicks to each side. After flutter kicking, bring legs together, then twist at the waist and move into sidestroke kick. Keep board flat on the surface, hands in position.
6. Flutter kick slowly as you count to 30 (one-half minute), then kick at a quicker pace for another half minute. Repeat several times and, as you practice, try to increase the duration of each pace to one minute. Also do this variation kicking on your back, or side, or while holding the pool rim as shown in Fig. 8-13.

FIGURE 8-13

7. Twist at the waist and flutter kick with the sides of your legs parallel to the surface. To do this, move your left hand down to grip the board when kicking on your right side (Fig. 8-7). Use the reverse hand position for the left side.
8. Kick forward while rolling over. Kick eight times on your front (Fig. 8-1) but with hands lower on board; then roll over and kick eight times on your back. Roll to your front and repeat the sequence across the pool. Keep board on the surface in front with hands in position. (Board will flip over as you roll.) To roll smoothly, (a) kick continuously and (b) when rolling to the right onto your back, start by pressing the right side of the board down. Kick eight times, then continue to roll in the same direction to your front by pressing the left side down. Reverse the process when rolling left. Practice rolling in both directions with face in or out of the water to exhale as you roll to your front. For variation, roll over without pausing to kick on your back. Instead, use eight kicks forward, then kick four times to roll over to the SP.

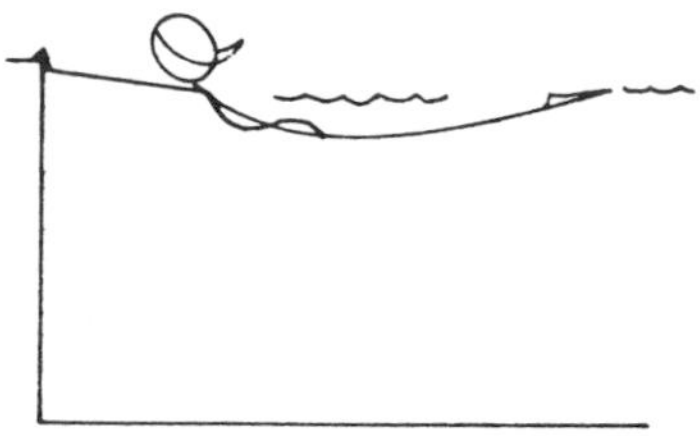

9. Kick while rolling as in #8, but this time swing the board in a circular pattern as you turn over, as in **Whirlabout** (p. 163). To do this, start as shown in Fig. 8-1. Then, as you roll to your back, swing the board along the surface to a position over your legs (Fig. 8-14). Roll to your front, swinging the board around to the SP. To roll smoothly, kick nonstop, swinging board with elbows straight. Practice rolling In both directions. For variety, kick without pausing on your back as in #8 variation while also swinging the board along the surface.

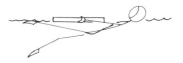

FIGURE 8-14

10. Hold the board on the surface in front and place both hands on top of it in the center. Now, kick fast, heels and head high, while pressing down against the board. This is very tiring, so intersperse some slower kicking. For variation, press down on the board with one hand and stroke "windmill" fashion with the other arm. Pull arm strongly through the water, all the way back, then circle it up and forward. Kick a set distance, then change to the other arm.
11. Flutter kick with your head up, holding the board crosswise on the surface behind, arms on top, fingers gripping outside edge (Fig. 8-15). Lift chin and press shoulder blades together.
12. Flutter kick from a vertical position while holding the board lightly on the surface in front (Fig. 8-16). Kick strongly and continuously to keep yourself high in the water. Vary by holding the board overhead or on top of your head. You also can use a breast stroke or sidestroke kick without the glide. You will stay in place for this variation.

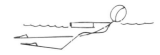

FIGURE 8-15

Flutter Kick Variations on Your Back. Hold board as in Fig. 8-2 but with chin tucked so that water level is along jaw and crown of head.

1. Kick quickly, flinging water into the air with your toes.
2. Kick slow to medium to fast (16 kicks at each speed).
3. Alternate 16 flutter kicks with 4 elementary backstroke kicks.
4. Keeping shoulders level, roll to your right hip. Now, flutter kick with legs parallel to the surface. Feel the stretch in waist, shoulders, and chest. Repeat on the left side.
5. Alternate flutter kick with sidestroke kick. Keep shoulders level and roll onto your right hip. Sidestroke kick two times moving top leg forward; roll to your back and flutter kick eight times. Repeat on the left side.
6. Raise the board overhead from the surface in back (Fig. 8-2) to the surface in front (Fig. 8-14). Alternate between the two positions while kicking strongly and continuously. Inhale as you raise the board to increase your buoyancy

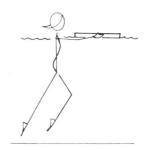

FIGURE 8-16

and keep face above the surface. Also try this version with a beach ball instead of a board.

7. Flutter kick backward with a bend at the hips.

a. Hold the board on the surface in front. From this position, bend at the hips to pike legs forward. Now, kick while trying to touch your toes to the board (Fig. 8-17). This kick will move you backward.

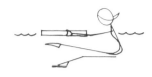

FIGURE 8-17

b. Kick while alternating between the positions shown in Figs. 8-14 and 8-17. Simply raise hips close to the surface, then lower them to the pike position, changing hip level every 16 kicks. Kick continuously, keeping elbows straight.

c. Kick while holding the board lengthwise against your back as in Fig. 8-18. Lean back at a 45° angle and position the board as needed for balance. Toes should reach the surface on the upward leg swing.

d. Hold the board crosswise behind with arms on top, fingers gripping back edge (Fig. 8-19). Bring toes to the surface on each upward kick. Strive to keep back and head erect.

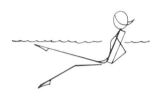

FIGURE 8-18

8. Start by kicking on your front and holding the board in back as in Fig. 8-15; then reverse direction by piking legs forward and kicking backward (Fig. 8-19). Kick nonstop as you change body position, keeping hands in place on the board. Alternate direction after each 16 kicks.

9. Flutter kick forward, holding the board as in Fig. 8-15; then roll to your back bringing legs into pike position (Fig. 8-20) and continue kicking in the same direction. Roll to your front and repeat the sequence across the pool. Kick nonstop as you roll over, keeping hands in place on the board. Kick 16 times in each position.

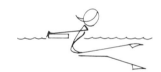

FIGURE 8-19

Breast Stroke Kick Variations

1. Kick slowly and sustain the glide. Stretch as you lift heels and press legs together. Hold the glide for a count of four.

2. On the propulsion phase of the kick (described in the basic breast stroke kick (#2, p. 141), push very forcefully with your feet for added thrust.

3. Kick fast, eliminating the glide entirely by pressing feet back forcefully but without bringing them together. Instead, immediately begin another kick, keeping feet flexed throughout. This version produces a strong, surging motion.

4. Alternate #1 with #3 above, using four kicks for each.

5. Alternate four breast stroke kicks with two sidestroke kicks to each side. After each kick, bring legs together and stretch/glide. Also, twist at the waist and keep shoulders level for the sidestroke kicks.

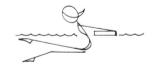

FIGURE 8-20

6. Kick and firm the muscles of your face at the same time. During breast stroke or flutter kicking, when you put your face down in the water to exhale, contract your face and neck muscles by using an exaggerated smile! Hold the contraction through your exhalation. Repeat 6 times, gradually increasing to 20.

7. Roll over by alternating four breast stroke kicks on your front with four elementary backstroke kicks on your back. Roll to your front again and repeat this sequence several times across the pool. Roll over as feet come together to glide, keeping board on the surface in front, hands in position. (Board will flip over as you roll.) Also practice turning in the opposite direction. As you roll to your front, head may be in or out of the water to exhale. To roll easily, start by pressing the right side of the board down when rolling right onto your back; then continue to roll in the same direction to your front by pressing the left side down. Reverse this process when rolling left.

Variations:

a. Omit the pause on your back by rolling completely over in one smooth motion. Kick four times on your front, then roll as you begin the glide portion of the fourth kick. To roll smoothly, put your face in the water to exhale and press down on one side of the board at the same time as instructed in #7 above. As you turn, stretch to streamline your body and keep legs together.

b. Kick and roll as suggested in #7 above, but instead of keeping the board forward, swing it along the surface as described in #9 of **Flutter Kick Variations on Your Front.** Even more variation is possible by rolling over in one smooth motion as in 7a above while also swinging the board along the surface.

Elementary Backstroke Kick Variations

1. Kick slowly and sustain the glide as you Tuck-in; stretch legs and press them tightly together. Hold for a count of six.

2. Kick fast and omit the glide as in #3 under **Breast Stroke Kick Variations.**

3. On the propulsion phase of the kick (described in #3, p. 142), push your feet forward with extra force for added thrust.

4. Alternate four slow kicks with four fast ones.

5. Alternate four elementary backstroke kicks with two sidestroke kicks to each side. Twist at the waist, keeping shoulders level during the side kicks. Practice some kicks moving the top leg forward and some moving it back.

Remember to bring legs together and stretch/glide after each kick.

6. Elementary backstroke kick with legs piked as in Fig. 8-17.

Sidestroke Kick Variations

1. Move your upper leg back instead of forward.
2. Move your upper leg alternately forward, then backward.
3. Extend the glide while counting to six. Inhale as feet come together to increase buoyancy and length of glide.
4. Use a flutter kick from the sidestroke position with legs parallel to and under the surface. Concentrate on a wide kick.
5. Combine sidestroke kick with flutter kick by alternating between 4 sidestroke kicks and 12 flutter kicks.
6. Repeat the variations listed above on the other side.

Aquabatics

At first glance, Kickboard Aquabatics may appear to be merely a whimsical diversion. While it's true that these Kapers are for the young at heart of any age, they nevertheless challenge one's balance, coordination, and agility—and, with a little practice, improve those skills. Moreover, they will refine posture and strengthen muscles of the trunk, arms, and hands and instill confidence in the water.

This section is divided into seven groups. Generally, each group of movements becomes more difficult. However, the degree of difficulty is subjective and depends to a large extent on your flexibility and coordination. Nonetheless, the ability to float on your front and back and recover to a standing position are prerequisites. Further, swimming skills are necessary for the **Flamingo** since it takes place in deeper water.

Aquabatics were developed to be used with an inexpensive styrofoam board approximately 12 × 22 × 1½ inches. Your favorite Aquabatics may be used along with other Aquacises in your workouts, or you can plan entire workouts using Aquabatics and Kickboarding as outlined in "Planning Your Water Workouts," Program B.

Aquabatics

CROCODILE (p. 150)
Pull Down in Front
Pull Down Side
Forward Push—Pull
Front Press Down—Lift
Press Down—Push Out
Arch—Tuck In
Leg Back—Arms Forward
Pull Down in Back
Extended Stretch
Backward Push—Pull
Back Press Down—Lift
Swing Tilt
Single Arm Press Down
Press Down—Swing Around
Push Side to Side
Press to Vertical

CLOWNFISH (p. 153)
Balance
Heels Back
Legs Forward
Knees Up
Knees Down
Cruise Forward or Backward
Turn Around
Double Arm and Knee Swing
Fingers to Toes
Sail the Seas
Circle the Globe

FLOUNDER (p. 155)
Balance
Lean Back
Tuck Knees
Pike Legs
Cruise Forward or Backward
Stretch Long on Back
Cruise Headfirst on Back
Cruise Foot First on Back
Hips Down—Hips Up
Scoop 'n Arch
Flip—Flop
Arch—Lean Back—Stretch Long
Balance with Feet Up

ANGELFISH (p. 158)
Legs High V-Split
Lift One Knee
Lift Both Knees
Knees Up—Swing Back
Swing To and Fro
Pedal
Boomerang

MOONFISH (p. 160)
Legs Side by Side
Legs High V-Split
Knees Up
Cruise Forward or Backward
Turn Around
Gentle Bounce
Split, Swing, 'n Touch

SWAN (p. 161)
Curve Up
Cruise Headfirst
Cruise Foot First
Cruise Back 'n Forth
Curve Up—Push Down
Curve Up—V-Split
One Knee Down
Both Knees Down
V-Split Front—V-Split Back
Legs Forward—Pull Back
Kneel
Whirlabout

FLAMINGO (p. 164)
Stand Up
Bend Up
Cruise Forward or Backward
Turn Around
Stand Up and Twist
Stand Up—Pivot—Bend Up
Stand Up—Curve Up—Push Down
One Leg Stand
Stand on One—Bend One
Stand on One—Extend One
Stand on One—Arc One
Cruise Forward or Backward

MORE KICKBOARD KAPERS (Ideas for Workouts, Games, and Races) (p. 166)

CROCODILE

Strengthens hands, arms, upper body; increases shoulder flexibility. Some movements add waist exercise

Each Kaper in this group consists of moving the kickboard against the water's resistance and is done while standing in the shallow water.

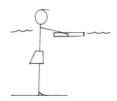

FIGURE 8-21

GET SET: Stand in shallow water at the depths suggested below. Feet should remain firmly on pool floor, so avoid water that is too deep.

GO: Choose a variety of Kapers from the following list and repeat each 10 to 20 times. Be sure to include forward, backward, and sideward arm movements.

Pull Down in Front. Stand in **chest-deep water** with your feet apart side to side. Hold the board crosswise in front at the surface, arms on top, fingers gripping the outside edge (Fig. 8-21). From this position, pull the board down to your legs, then lift it to the SP. To increase resistance, hold the board by each end. Keep elbows straight.

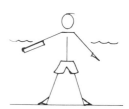

FIGURE 8-22

Pull Down Side. Stand in **chest-deep water** with your feet apart side to side. Hold the board out to one side with your arm on top, fingers gripping the outside edge (Fig. 8-22). Now, press down on the board, then lift it up to the start. After several repetitions, perform with the other arm. You also can do this with a board under each arm.

Forward Push—Pull. Stand in **chest-deep water,** feet apart front to back, knees bent. Hold the board half submerged and by each end in front of your chest, elbows straight (board perpendicular to the floor, Fig. 8-23). Now, briskly pull the board toward your chest then push it forward to the start. For greater difficulty, perform with the board completely submerged. Or, use two boards, one on top of the other with edges overlapped.

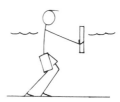

FIGURE 8-23

Front Press Down—Lift. Stand in **chest-deep water,** feet apart side to side. Hold the board by each end at the surface in front of your chest, elbows bent (Fig. 8-24). From this position, press it straight down (straightening elbows), then lift it up to the start. Press and lift rapidly. For more resistance, hold two boards, one on top of the other with edges overlapped. For *variation,* alternate this movement with **Forward Push—Pull.**

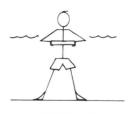

FIGURE 8-24

Press Down—Push Out. Stand in **chest-deep water,** feet apart front to back. Hold the board by each end at the surface close to your chest, elbows bent. Now, press the board straight down (straightening elbows), then push it forward and up to the surface (Fig. 8-25). Reverse the motion and return to the SP.

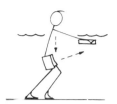

FIGURE 8-25

Arch—Tuck-In. Perform **Press Down—Push Out** with your feet apart side to side. This time, arch your back as you push the board forward (Fig. 8-26). Return to the start by pushing it down toward your legs as you Tuck-in and press hips back (Fig. 8-27).

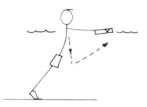

FIGURE 8-26

Leg Back—Arms Forward. Do **Press Down—Push Out** starting with feet together. As arms move down and forward, lift one leg to the back. Hold the stretch for eight counts by lifting head, chest, and leg as you press down slightly on the board for leverage (Fig. 8-28). Next, tip head forward, Tuck-in, and return to the start. Alternate legs.

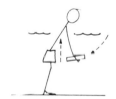

FIGURE 8-27

Pull Down in Back. Stand in **waist-deep water** with feet apart side to side. Hold the board flat against your backside, arms on top, fingers gripping the outside edge. Tuck-in to stabilize yourself. Now, lift the board up to the back (Fig. 8-29) then pull it down to the start. For greater resistance, hold the board by each end. Keep elbows straight.

Extended Stretch. Use the same SP as **Pull Down in Back.** Now, lift the board up to the back, then slowly lean back to the limit of your shoulder flexibility (Fig. 8-30). Relax chest and shoulders and hold for a slow count of eight, then pull yourself upright, relax, and repeat a total of three times.

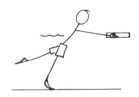

FIGURE 8-28

Backward Push—Pull. Stand in **waist-deep water** with feet apart side to side. Grasp each end of the board with elbows bent and hold it half submerged with the flat surface against your hips in back (Fig. 8-31). Now, push the board straight back (straightening elbows), then pull it to the start keeping board perpendicular.

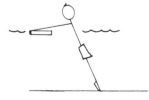

FIGURE 8-30

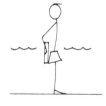

FIGURE 8-31

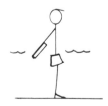

FIGURE 8-29

Back Press Down—Lift. Stand in **waist-deep water** with feet apart side to side. Hold the board by each end behind your back, elbows bent. Place the forward edge close to your back, the flat surface parallel with the pool floor. Now, press the board straight down (straightening elbows), then lift it to the start (Fig. 8-32). Press and lift briskly. For variation, alternate this movement with **Backward Push—Pull.**

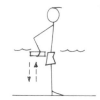

FIGURE 8-32

Swing Tilt. (Adds waist exercise.) Stand in **waist-deep water** with feet apart side to side. Hold the board in front at the surface, palms on top. Now, swing it through the surface as you twist from side to side. Press down harder with one hand to tilt the board in the direction of motion (Fig. 8-33).

Single Arm Press Down. Stand in **waist-deep water,** feet apart side to side. Hold the board at the surface in front, one hand placed in the center. Now, push the board straight down (Fig. 8-34) then let it rise slowly. Periodically change to the other arm.

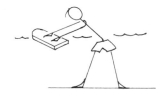

FIGURE 8-33

Press Down—Swing Around. Perform **Single Arm Press Down** but, before letting board rise to the surface, swing it around to the back. (Keep it close to your leg, elbow straight.) Swing board to the front again and let it rise to the start. Repeat with the other arm.

Push Side to Side. (Adds waist exercise). Stand in **waist-deep water,** feet apart side to side. Hold the board perpendicular to the pool floor in front of your chest, elbows bent. Place one hand in the center of each side (Fig. 8-35). Now, swing the board from side to side. The deeper you submerge the board, the greater the resistance. Keep stomach pulled in.

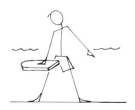

FIGURE 8-34

Press to Vertical. Stand in **waist-deep water** with feet apart side to side. Hold the board by its inside edge at the surface in front. Now, using your hands and wrists, press down until the board is vertical (Figs. 8-36 and 8-37) then let it rise to the start.

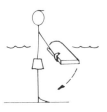

FIGURE 8-36

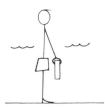

FIGURE 8-37

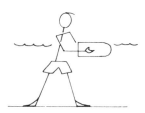

FIGURE 8-35

CLOWNFISH

Strengthens arms, upper body, and abdomen; increases flexibility of shoulders and chest; improves posture

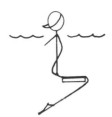

FIGURE 8-38

During this group of Kapers, you will sit atop the kickboard, then move forward and backward using your arms. You'll also turn around or swing your legs from side to side. Then, for an encore, you can somersault with the board locked behind your knees.

GET SET: Stand in the shallow water and hold the board by each end behind your back. Now, pull it under your thighs, as if pulling up a chair, and sit on it. Position its forward edge just behind your knees and sit with knees either apart or together.

GO: To develop balance and control, first learn to balance on the board with your legs in the various positions given below. Keep head and back erect, stomach pulled in. This will prepare you for the remaining **Clownfish** movements.

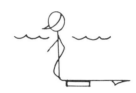

FIGURE 8-39

Balance Heels Back. Balance on the board with knees facing forward, heels pressed back to hold the board securely (Fig. 8-38). Balance with arms out to each side, hands at the surface, palms down.

Balance Legs Forward. Balance with legs forward, and knees straight. Hold arms out to each side, with hands at the surface, palms down (Fig. 8-39).

Balance Knees Up. Balance with knees together and lifted toward your chest (Fig. 8-40), arms either forward or out to each side. This version, while difficult at first, is especially effective for firming your abdomen.

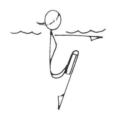

FIGURE 8-40

Balance Knees Down. Balance with knees down, heels pressed toward your buttocks and with arms either forward or sideward, hands at the surface, palms down (Fig. 8-41). This Kaper will help to firm your buttocks and the back of your thighs.

Cruise Forward or Backward. Use your arms as described in **Oarfish** arm motion (p. 27) to move forward or backward across the pool with your legs in each of the previously described balance positions.

Turn Around. Now, try turning around with knees in each balance position. You can turn by pulling inward with one arm, then immediately press outward with the other arm, hands just under the surface. Or, pull inward with one arm while keeping

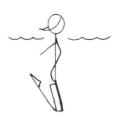

FIGURE 8-41

the other hand on your hip. See if you can turn in a full circle with just two forceful pulls. Periodically change to the other arm and turn in the opposite direction.

Double Arm and Knee Swing. (Adds waist exercise.) With legs in each of the balance positions, swing arms and knees from side to side opposite to one another. Start with arms out to each side, then move the left arm across in front as you swing the right arm back. Reverse the motion, swinging arms forward to the left. Swing smoothly and continuously until stomach or arm muscles become fatigued. Keep hands close to the surface, palms tilted in the direction of movement (Fig. 8-42).

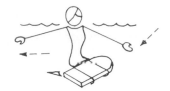

FIGURE 8-42

Fingers to Toes. Sit erect with arms sideward at the surface and with legs forward, either apart or together, knees straight (Fig. 8-39). Now, lift your legs as you swing arms forward, touching fingers to toes (Fig. 8-43). Return to the SP and repeat 8 to 20 times with a rhythmic, bouncing motion. Keep knees straight, feet extended, and stomach pulled in. If feet are lifted too high, the board may slide out of position, so always reach far forward.

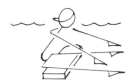

FIGURE 8-43

Sail the Seas. Sit crosswise on the board with the left knee straight, right knee bent to lock the board securely against upper thigh (Fig. 8-44). Now, move forward across the pool using **Oarfish** arm motion (p. 27). Next, turn your trunk 180° to the right. As you do, rotate at the left hip joint, keeping left leg elevated, knee straight. You now face your starting point with the left leg extended back (Fig. 8-45). Finally, you can either (1) reverse the 180° turn and continue stroking forward across the pool, (2) stroke backward across the pool using the **Reverse Oarfish** arm motion (p. 27), or (3) stroke forward to your starting point. Periodically switch to the right leg forward and turn to the left. For smooth coordination, turn around when arms have moved back to shoulder level. Use a small inward pull with one hand (right hand when turning right, etc.). Lift your chest and the heel of the extended leg.

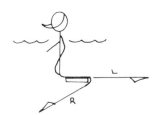

FIGURE 8-44

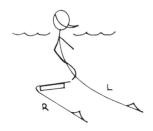

FIGURE 8-45

Circle the Globe. Somersault forward or backward starting from any of the previously described balanced sitting positions. If coordination is difficult in the beginning, practice arm movements alone while standing in the shallow water. Remember to stay tightly tucked until body has turned a complete revolution.

Circle South. Tuck chin down and lift knees toward your forehead. At the same time, rotate arms in a "down-back-up-forward" circle, elbows straight (Fig. 8-46). One or two arm

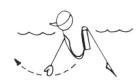

FIGURE 8-46

circles should easily somersault you backward around to the SP. When you can somersault once and return to the start, try it two or three times in succession, catching a breath each time you pass the SP.

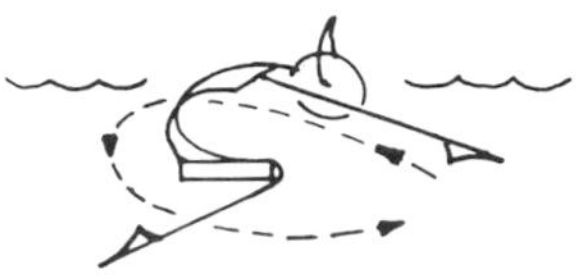

FIGURE 8-47

Circle North. Simultaneously tuck chin down and reach arms forward and down. Now, somersault forward by rotating arms in an "up-back-down-forward" direction, elbows straight (Fig. 8-47). The hardest part of this Kaper is returning to the upright SP so you will need to continue to press arms in the same direction but with extra force.

Note: During front and back somersaults, either exhale through your nose or wear a nose clip.

FLOUNDER

Strengthens arms, upper body, and abdomen; increases trunk and shoulder flexibility

This group of Aquabatics will especially challenge your balance and coordination. Starting from an upright sitting position on the board, you'll move into other sitting and back-floating positions with the board under your calves. Movements in this group utilize body positions ranging from tuck to pike to arch.

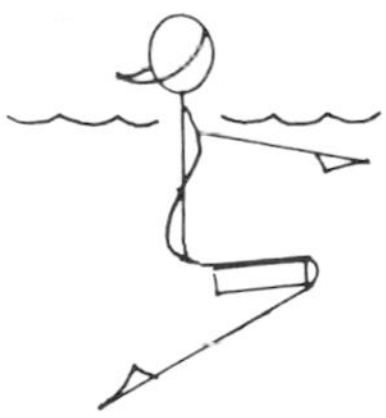

FIGURE 8-48

GET SET: Sit with the board crosswise under your thighs with the forward edge just behind your knees. Press heels back to hold it securely (Fig. 8-48). Extend arms forward in a V-position (halfway between forward and sideward), hands close to the surface.

GO: Practice balancing in the following positions, holding each for a few seconds with hands at the surface, back straight, and stomach in. (As you lift legs to move into position, the board will float up under your calves.) Recover to the SP, as instructed below, and repeat each position several times before moving to the next. This will prepare you for the other Aquabatics in this group.

To recover to the start with the board again under your thighs, press heels down and tip head forward while forcefully rotating arms as in **Circle North** above. The firm pressure of your lower legs against the board will flip it back under your thighs.

Balance Lean Back. From the **Get Set** position, lean back and lift knees until board flips under calves as shown in Fig. 8-49. Edge of board should be directly behind heels to lock it in place. Keep head in line with body, feet extended, toes at the surface.

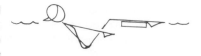

FIGURE 8-49

Balance Tuck Knees. From the **Get Set** position, lift knees toward chest, letting board float into position under your calves with the front edge directly behind your heels. Keep trunk erect (Fig. 8-50).

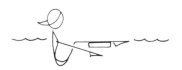

FIGURE 8-50

Balance Pike Legs. From the **Get Set** position, lean back and let the board float into position under your calves with the front edge directly behind heels. Next, straighten knees and pike sharply (Fig. 8-51).

Cruise Forward or Backward. Use your arms as described in **Oarfish** (p. 27) to move forward or backward across the pool with your body in each of the balance positions above.

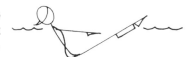

FIGURE 8-51

Stretch Long on Back. Start from any of the three balance positions (board under calves), then stretch out to your back with head in line with spine, eyes looking straight up (Fig. 8-52). Recover to the SP. Start with 8 and work up to 20 repetitions.

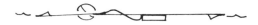

FIGURE 8-52

Cruise Headfirst on Back. To travel across the pool in a headfirst direction while in **Stretch Long** position, start with hands next to hips. Bend elbows and slide hands up the sides of your body to a position overhead; turn palms out and pull arms down to the start, elbows straight. Hands remain under the surface.

Cruise Foot First on Back. To travel across the pool in a foot first direction in **Stretch Long** position, start with hands next to hips, palms facing up. Scoop hands overhead, thumbs leading the way, elbows straight. Then, bend elbows and slide hands down sides of body to hips. Keep hands under the surface.

Hips Down—Hips Up. Start in the **Balance Legs Forward** position (Fig. 8-53). Keeping board under thighs, lean back into **Stretch Long** as you scoop arms sideward and overhead

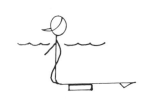

FIGURE 8-53

(hands just under the surface, palms facing up, elbows straight, Fig. 8-52). Return to the upright SP by sharply lowering your hips and scooping arms down and forward. Alternate between sitting and lying positions moving smoothly from one to the other. Start with 8 and work up to 20 repetitions.

Remember: (1) Stretch and tense legs and extend feet. (2) Pull in stomach hard when lowering hips to sit upright. (3) Stretch to your limit from fingers to toes when in **Stretch Long.**

Scoop 'n Arch. Perform **Hips Down—Hips Up** as suggested. However, this time as you move into **Stretch Long,** arch your back and submerge your head and trunk (Fig. 8-54). Use arms to assist by forcefully pressing them down and overhead as you tip head back and arch. Reverse arm motion and return to the SP. For variation, perform **Scoop 'n Arch** from the **Balance Pike Legs** position with the board under calves as in Fig. 8-51.

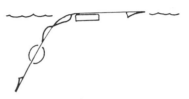

FIGURE 8-54

Remember: (1) Keep hands under the surface. (2) To arch, stretch from head to extended feet, lift chest, and tighten buttocks. (3) Keep stomach pulled in. (4) To avoid getting water in your nose, wear a nose clip or exhale continuously through your nose while your face is under water.

Flip—Flop. Start in the **Get Set** position (board under thighs) and lean back into **Stretch Long** (Fig. 8-55). From this position, lower hips and bend knees toward chest until the board flips under your calves (Fig. 8-56). Stretch out again (Fig. 8-57), then bend knees and push heels down until board flops back into position under your thighs (Fig. 8-58). **Flip—Flop** several times before returning to the upright SP. Then, do the sequence again!

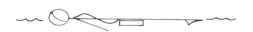

FIGURE 8-55

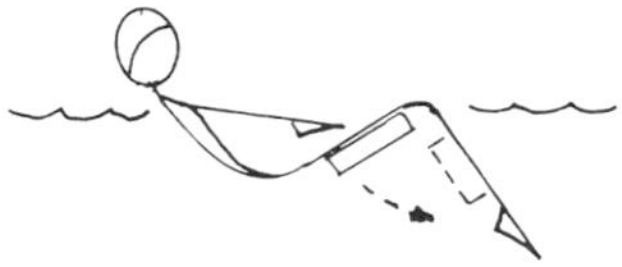

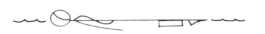

FIGURE 8-57

FIGURE 8-56

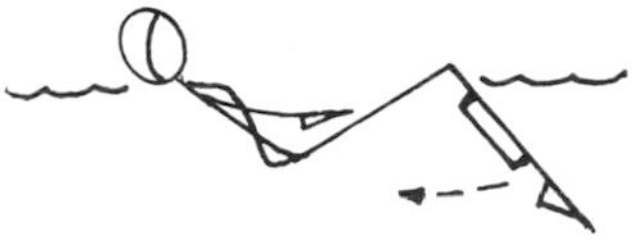

FIGURE 8-58

Arch—Lean Back—Stretch Long. From the **Get Set** position (Fig. 8-59), press knees down and arch your back until feet surface behind (Fig. 8-60). Immediately roll over into **Lean Back** balance position (board will flip under calves, Fig. 8-61), then **Stretch Long** (Fig. 8-62).

To return to the upright SP, bend knees and hips into **Lean Back.** Then, either

1. Tip forward by pressing heels back and scooping arms as in **Circle North** (p. 155). Board will flip into position under thighs as you press heels back and sit up.
2. Roll over and arch (Fig. 8-60) then scoop arms as in **Circle South** (p. 154) as you tuck knees forward.

    Remember to maintain firm control over your stomach muscles, especially as you arch, to avoid excessive hyperextension of the lower back.

Balance with Feet Up. To stretch your back, start from **Balance Tuck Knees** position (Fig. 8-50) then grasp the board by each end. Turn it perpendicular to pool floor. Now, place the soles of both feet in the center, feet together (Fig. 8-63), and balance for several seconds; then return to the SP. To vary, start from the position shown in Fig. 8-63. Now, alternately extend legs straight down to vertical, then lift feet up to the SP. Perform briskly 10 to 30 times.

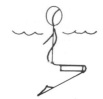

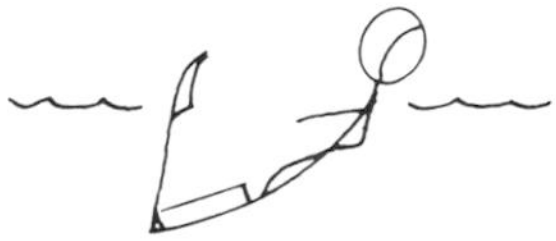

FIGURE 8-59

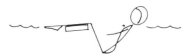

FIGURE 8-60

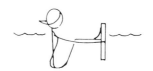

FIGURE 8-61

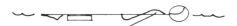

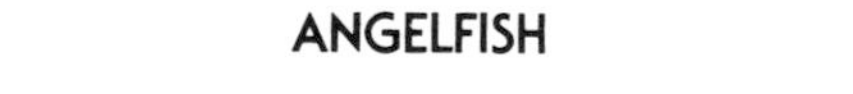

FIGURE 8-62

ANGELFISH

Balancing stunts strengthen muscles of the trunk—both fore and aft—while brisk leg movements tone muscles of the legs

This group of Kapers will challenge your coordination and ability to balance in various ways while suspending yourself over the board.

GET SET: Sit on the kickboard while holding it sideways by each end, legs together, knees straight. Press board straight down and balance (Fig. 8-64). To maintain balance, experiment with trunk vertical, slightly forward, or back.

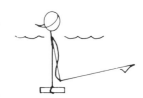

FIGURE 8-63

FIGURE 8-64

GO: Learn the first five **Angelfish** movements separately, then move through the entire group in sequence, performing each several times. Change position slowly and return to the SP after each change. For best control, pull in your stomach firmly. The remaining two **Angelfish** use brisk leg movements and may be used whenever you can balance in the positions shown in Figs. 8-64 and 8-68.

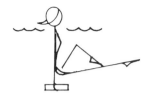

FIGURE 8-65

Legs High V-Split. From the **Get Set** position, separate legs into a high, wide V-split, keeping knees straight and feet extended.

Lift One Knee. Lift knees alternately toward chest (Fig. 8-65).

Lift Both Knees. Tuck up both knees simultaneously toward chest (Fig. 8-66).

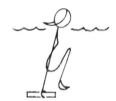

FIGURE 8-66

Knees Up—Swing Back. Keeping legs together, tuck up both knees, then swing legs to the back (Figs. 8-67 and 8-68). Reverse the movement by tucking up knees, then extend legs forward to the SP.

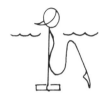

FIGURE 8-67

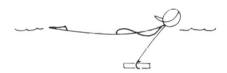

FIGURE 8-68

Swing To and Fro. With knees and elbows straight, press hips back and swing the board under your legs toward your heels (Fig. 8-69). Then press hips forward and swing the board back (Fig. 8-70). Keep flat surface of the board parallel with the floor. For better balance, separate legs.

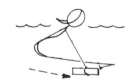

FIGURE 8-69

Pedal. Hold the board sideways by each end and sit with your hips either on, or forward of, the board. Now, travel forward across the pool while pedaling an imaginary bicycle (Fig. 8-71). Pedal strongly with feet flexed or extended. Reach your feet far forward, then press them down and back against the water. Keep back straight. Also turn around by pedaling four times for each 360° turn. To vary, try several sequences of the following: pedal forward 8 times; then, without changing body position, flutter kick backward 16 times to your starting point. When moving in either direction, cover as much distance as possible and maintain that same distance in subsequent repetitions.

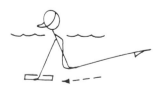

FIGURE 8-70

Boomerang. Suspend yourself in the position shown in Fig. 8-64. Now, open legs sideward to a wide V-split, then close them forcefully. Repeat briskly 10 to 30 times, keeping feet extended and close to the surface.

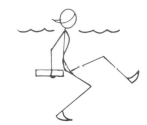

FIGURE 8-71

MOONFISH

Strengthens abdomen, arms, and upper body

This group of Aquabatics also will challenge your ability to balance on the board—this time on the end of your spine. Your abdominal muscles will work hard to hold you in position.

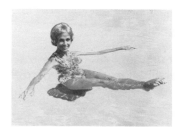

FIGURE 8-72

GET SET: Sit on the board. (Try sitting with the board crosswise or lengthwise.) Pull in your stomach.

GO: First, learn to balance motionless. (In the beginning, you may need to move hands gently under the surface to maintain equilibrium.) This gets you ready to move about the pool using your arms as in **Cruise Forward** or **Backward.** Then, for other challenges, try **Gentle Bounce** and **Swing Side—Crossover.**

Legs Side by Side. Lean back as required to bring your legs into a pike position with toes at the surface. Hold hands at the surface, palms down, with arms sideward or forward. Keep your back straight and stomach in. Stretch your legs and extend your feet (Fig. 8-72).

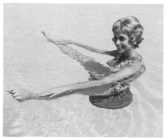

FIGURE 8-73

Legs High V-Split. Balance with legs and arms separated in a wide V, knees and elbows straight (Fig. 8-73). Pull in your stomach and extend your feet with toes at the surface.

Knees Up. Balance with knees bent, toes at the surface, and with thighs perpendicular to the floor. Hold arms either sideward or forward (Fig. 8-74).

Cruise Forward or **Backward.** Stroke arms gently to move forward or backward across the pool using the **Oarfish** arm motion described on p. 27.

Turn Around. To turn in either direction, pull lightly toward yourself with one arm, then immediately press outward with the other arm, hands just under the surface.

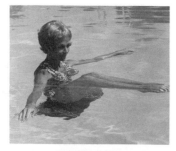

FIGURE 8-74

Gentle Bounce. Bounce up and down by raising and lowering arms at the side as in **Butterflyfish** (p. 26). Keep hands under the surface and legs in **Legs Side by Side** or **High V-Split** position. Hips remain in contact with the board.

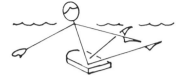

FIGURE 8-75

Split, Swing 'n Touch. (Adds waist exercise.) Start with arms sideward, legs in a high V-split. Now, swing arms and legs from side to side opposite to one another, crossing over to touch hand to opposite foot (Fig. 8-75). To swing arms, move one arm across in front as you swing the other back, keeping hands close to the surface, palms tilted in the direction of motion.

SWAN

Strengthens all muscles of the trunk, particularly the back, buttocks, and abdomen. Also increases flexibility of the trunk, while arm movements strengthen arms, upper trunk

The Kapers in the first part of this group are performed while lying front down on the board. Those in the second part are performed lying front down, but with the board held beneath your body at arms' length. From this position, you will use your legs in a variety of ways. Lastly, you will swing the board in a circle at the surface while rolling over.

GET SET: Experiment to position the board lengthwise under your abdomen so that it stays in place.

GO: Start by learning to balance on the board in **Curve Up** position, then move one by one through the entire group until you have mastered them all. Keep stomach pulled in, legs stretched, and feet extended.

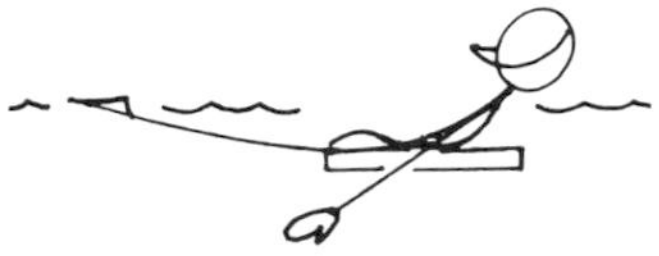

Curve Up. Balance on the board with arms at your sides, head and heels lifted to arch your back (Fig. 8-76). Stretch legs, tighten buttocks, and press shoulders back.

FIGURE 8-76

Cruise Headfirst. Start in the **Curve Up** position, but with arms forward and straight, palms turned outward. Now, forcefully pull arms out to each side and all the way back to your hips. Next, bend elbows and slide hands close to your body and up to the SP. Keep hands under the surface as you pull yourself across the pool.

Cruise Foot First. Reverse headfirst arm motion and forcefully scoop arms forward. Start with arms straight and at your sides;

then, with palms facing forward, scoop arms forward until palms touch. Bend elbows and slide hands close to your body down to the start. Always keep hands under the surface.

Cruise Back 'n Forth. From **Curve Up** position, stroke 10 times headfirst then stroke 10 times in a foot first direction. Repeat the sequence three or more times.

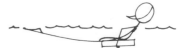
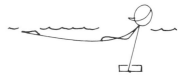

FIGURE 8-77

Curve Up—Push Down. Begin in **Curve Up** position, but this time hold the board crosswise by each end against your midsection (Fig. 8-77). Now, press the board down until elbows are straight (Fig. 8-78). Balance with heels lifted, chest up, legs straight and together. Return to this position after each repetition of the following six Kapers. Move slowly to maintain balance while keeping stomach pulled in.

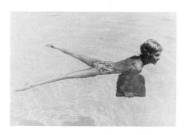

FIGURE 8-78

Curve Up—V-Split. From **Curve Up—Push Down** position, separate legs into a wide V-split (Fig. 8-79), then close legs together. Move extra slowly, keeping buttocks tight, legs stretched, and heels lifted to the surface. Start with 10 and work up to 20 repetitions.

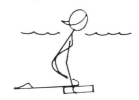

FIGURE 8-79

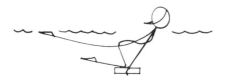

FIGURE 8-80

One Knee Down. From **Curve Up—Push Down** position, move one knee down to the board while keeping the other leg extended, heel lifted, chest up (Fig. 8-80). Move leg slowly up to the SP and repeat, alternating legs. Start with 8 repetitions for each leg and work up to 15.

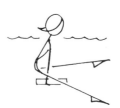

FIGURE 8-81

Both Knees Down. From **Curve Up—Push Down** position, bend knees and move them down to the board (Fig. 8-81); then straighten legs slowly back to the start. Start with 10 and work up to 20 repetitions.

V-Split Front—V-Split Back. From **Curve Up—Push Down** position, separate legs to a wide V-split, then swing them forward as you move trunk to an upright position, legs in a wide V-split (Fig. 8-82). Reverse the action and swing legs back to the start. Keep feet extended, legs stretched and separated as far as

FIGURE 8-82

possible as you change position. Start with 10 and work up to 20 repetitions. Also try this one holding the board lengthwise by each side.

Legs Forward—Pull Back. From **Curve Up—Push Down,** pike at the hips and swing feet down and forward, legs together. At the same time, bend elbows and pull the board toward your midsection (Fig. 8-83). Then return to the SP by pressing board straight down and lifting legs up to the back. For variation, bend knees to move legs forward; straighten them briefly, then bend them again before lifting them back to the start. Begin with 8 repetitions and gradually work up to 15.

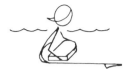
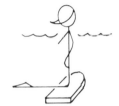

FIGURE 8-83

Kneel. Start in **Curve Up—Push Down** position. Now, bend both knees and kneel on the board. Balance with arms sideward (Fig. 8-84) or travel around the pool using the **Oarfish** arm motion (p. 27).

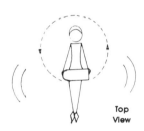

FIGURE 8-84

Whirlabout: Swing the board in a circle on the surface of the water. Start on your back, holding the board by each end and positioned over your thighs with elbows straight (Fig. 8-85). Now, (1) swing the board to the left and roll over to your left side at the same time, Fig. 8-86, (2) swing board overhead and roll to your front, Fig. 8-87, (3) swing board around to the right and roll onto right side, Fig. 8-88, (4) swing board down to the start and roll to your back. **Whirlabout** three times to each side, moving smoothly and continuously. Repeat this sequence two or more times.

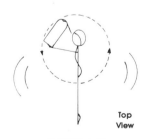

FIGURE 8-85

Remember: (1) Tuck-in and stretch from head to toe, keeping feet extended and together. (2) Keep elbows straight. (3) To help roll over, swing board energetically, keeping it on the surface. (4) Hold head in line with body, tipping it back if necessary to keep face dry when rolling to your front.

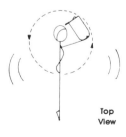

FIGURE 8-86

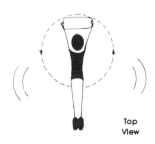

FIGURE 8-87

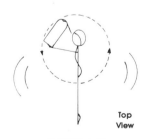

FIGURE 8-88

FLAMINGO

Tones body and improves posture, balance,
and coordination

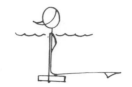

FIGURE 8-89

In this final group of Kapers, you'll learn to stand on the board in various ways. This may seem impossible at first, but even children can master these Aquabatics with a little determination.

GET SET: Start in calm water deep enough so that you can stand on the board while it floats freely. Hold it sideways by each end in either of the positions shown in Figs. 8-89 or 8-90.

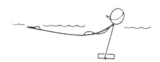

FIGURE 8-90

GO: Before doing the arm movements, learn to balance on the board. Then, build on your skills by adding the remaining movements. For best control, avoid water turbulence by changing position slowly. In the beginning, you may find yourself careening helplessly in one direction while the board sails off in the other. When you begin to lose control, bend your knees and quickly grab the board to keep it from zooming into someone close by. Then, start over again.

Stand Up. From the **Get Set** position, bend knees and place feet on the board. Feet can be together, apart, or turned out with toes curled over the ends of the board. Next, slowly straighten legs until you are standing. Later, try standing on the balls of your feet (Fig. 8-91). Hands may be used under the surface for gentle paddling or sculling. However, keep this to a minimum and rely primarily on good body alignment for balance. (Tuck-in tightly, lift chest with head erect.)

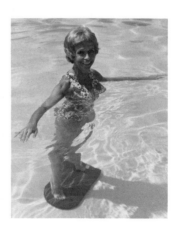

FIGURE 8-91

Bend Up. From **Stand Up** position, alternately bend and straighten legs (Fig. 8-92). Keep back erect. Repeat 10 to 20 times.

Cruise Forward or Backward. Travel about the pool while in **Stand Up** or **Bend Up** positions. Use arms as in **Oarfish** (p. 27).

Turn Around. You can turn by pulling inward with one arm, then immediately pressing outward with the other, hands just under the surface.

Stand Up and Twist. From **Stand Up** position, rotate hips from side to side while swinging arms in opposition (that is, turn hips left as you swing arms right). Start with arms out to each side, then move left arm across in front as you move the right arm

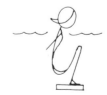

FIGURE 8-92

back. Reverse the motion, swinging arms around to the left. Swing smoothly and continuously, keeping hands close to the surface, palms tilted in the direction of motion (Fig. 8-93). Start with 8 repetitions to each side and work up to 15.

Stand Up—Pivot—Bend Up. Stand on the balls of your feet (Fig. 8-91). Now, pivot to the left (Fig. 8-94), then bend knees sharply and balance for several seconds (Fig. 8-95). Stand and repeat to the right. Repeat 5 to 10 times to each side.

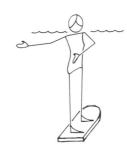

FIGURE 8-93

Stand Up—Curve Up—Push Down. From the **Stand Up** position, bend knees and grasp the board by each end; then push board down and extend legs to the back (Fig. 8-90). Next, bend knees, place feet on the board, and stand. Start with 10 repetitions and work up to 20.

One Leg Stand. Hold the board lengthwise, hands gripping each side. From the prone position shown in Fig. 8-90, bend knees and place one foot in the center of the board. Now, slowly straighten your leg until you are standing upright (Fig. 8-96). (Later, try standing on the ball of your foot.) Bend knees and grasp board as you return to the prone position. Repeat by alternating legs.

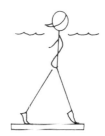

FIGURE 8-94

Stand on One—Bend One. Start by standing on one leg, then bend the other knee, keeping your toes in contact with the supporting leg (Fig. 8-97). Now, pull yourself forward across the pool.

Stand on One—Extend One. Start in **Stand Up** position. First, lift one leg high to the front (Fig. 8-98), then press it down to the start. Next, lift leg to side and return; then to the back and return. To lift leg back, lean far forward from the hip and lift heel up to the surface. Do the sequence three or more times before repeating with the other leg. Keep knees straight.

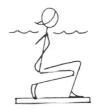

FIGURE 8-95

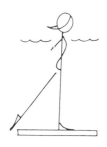

FIGURE 8-96

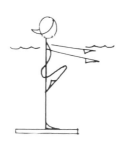

FIGURE 8-97

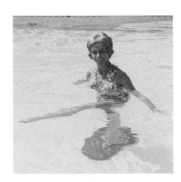

FIGURE 8-98

Stand on One—Arc One. Stand on one leg while slowly swinging the other in a wide arc. First, bring leg forward, then out to the side and around to the back. Keep knees straight and swing leg as high as possible. Repeat 5 to 10 times with each leg.

Cruise Forward or Backward. Use your arms to travel forward or backward across the pool while in **One Leg Stand, Stand on One—Bend One,** or **Stand on One—Extend One** (to the front, side or back, Fig. 8-99). Use arms **Oarfish** style as described on p. 27.

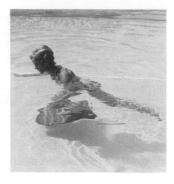

FIGURE 8-99

Flamingo is the final challenge to your balancing prowess—almost. While developing these movements, I concluded that if one can balance on the board while right-side-up, one could also balance upside down. I couldn't do it, but maybe you can.

More Kickboard Kapers
(Ideas for Workouts, Games, and Races)

To add more fun to your workouts and to increase your fitness level as well, move back and forth across the pool with these combined movements from the "Aquabatics," "Kickboarding," and the "Walk, Jog, Jump, Hop, and Kick" sections. Use them in your workouts as racing games (across two to four widths of the pool) or to improve your cardiovascular fitness (by moving slower and farther).

The idea is to move across the pool using one style of locomotion then return using another. You can use your arms to pull across while you sit, stand, kneel, or lie on the board; then return using your legs to kick, run, walk, etc., while holding the board. Workouts can be even more challenging if you stop along the way to jump in various ways or to balance on the board. These and other ideas have been incorporated in the following suggestions. However, to get off to a good start when racing, practice the upcoming movements before-hand.

IDEAS FROM CLOWNFISH AQUABATICS

1. Move back and forth across the pool using **Cruise Forward** or **Cruise Backward** arm movements (p. 153) while sitting in **Heels Back, Legs Forward, Knees Up, Knees Down,** or **Sail the**

Seas positions. Or, move across in one position and return in another.

2. Stop midway and repeat any of the following several times: **Turn Around, Double Arm and Knee Swing, Fingers to Toes,** or **Circle the Globe.**

3. **Cruise Forward** to the center of the pool while sitting in any of the positions suggested in #1; then, turn 180° and continue across the pool backward, using **Cruise Backward** arm motion.

4. During a workout (not a race), see how few **Cruise Forward** or **Cruise Backward** strokes you need to get across the pool. Pull arms forcefully, constantly striving for the smallest number.

IDEAS FROM FLOUNDER AQUABATICS

1. Move across the pool using **Cruise Forward** or **Backward** arm movements while in **Lean Back, Tuck Knees,** or **Pike Legs** positions. Or, move across in one position, return in another.

2. Stop midway to **Turn Around** once In each direction or turn halfway around, then continue backward across the pool using **Cruise Backward** arm motion.

3. Move across the pool in **Stretch Long** position, using arms as in **Cruise Headfirst on Back** and **Cruise Foot First** (p. 156). Stop midway and repeat six times any of the following: **Hips Down—Hips Up, Scoop 'n Arch, Flip—Flop,** or **Balance with Feet Up** variation, performing it briskly.

4. Alternate **Stretch Long** with **Lean Back, Tuck,** or **Pike** balance positions while cruising head or foot first across the pool. Stroke continuously and change from one body position to the other every six strokes.

5. From the **Get Set** position, use the **Cruise Forward** arm motion to move to the center of the pool. Then, either (a) assume the position shown in Fig. 8-60 and continue to stroke across the pool or (b) move into **Arch—Lean Back—Stretch Long** and continue across using **Cruise Headfirst** arm motion.

IDEAS FROM SWAN AQUABATICS

1. **Cruise Headfirst** across the pool in **Curve Up** position, then return in **Kneel.** Or, move forward in either position, then return moving backward using the reverse arm motion.

2. **Cruise Headfirst** across the pool, body in **Curve Up** position. Stop midway and repeat **Cruise Back 'n Forth** several times.

3. **Cruise Headfirst** across the pool in **Curve Up** or **Kneel.** Pause in the center and move into **Curve Up—Push Down.** From

this position, repeat any of the following eight times: **V-Split, One Knee Down, Both Knees Down, V-Split Front—V-Split Back, Legs Forward—Pull Back,** or **Whirlabout.** (Repeat four times in each direction. Move right into the first circle by rolling to your back (Fig. 8-85); then, after the eighth one, end on your front and push arms down to **Curve Up— Push Down.**)

4. Start from the position shown in Fig. 8-78. Now, perform four **One Knee Down** or **Both Knees Down** movements. Next, with legs back in the SP, flutter or breast stroke kick forward 18 times. Repeat the sequence across the pool.

5. Perform **Legs Forward—Pull Back.** When legs are forward, flutter kick backward 16 times; when legs are back, flutter kick forward 32 times. Repeat this sequence across the pool.

6. Use eight **Cruise Forward** arm strokes while in **Kneel** position, then grasp the ends of the board. Push board straight down and extend legs back to **Curve Up—Push Down** position (Fig. 8-78). Flutter or breast stroke kick forward 16 kicks. Bring knees foward and **Kneel** again, then repeat the sequence across the pool.

7. Perform **V-Split Front—V-Split Back.** Then, with legs extended to the back (Fig. 8-78), flutter or breast stroke kick forward 16 times. Repeat the sequence across the pool.

IDEAS FROM FLAMINGO AQUABATICS

1. Move across the pool using **Cruise Forward** or **Cruise Backward** arm strokes while in **Stand Up, Bend Up, One Leg Stand, Stand on One—Bend One,** or **Stand on One—Extend One** position. Pull arms smoothly to avoid turbulence that could swamp you.

2. Stop on the way and perform six repetitions of one or more of the following: **Stand Up and Twist, Turn Around** (three times in each direction), **Stand Up—Pivot—Bend Up, Stand Up—Curve Up—Push Down,** or **Stand on One—Arc One** (three times with each leg). Then, **Cruise Forward** or **Backward** across the pool in a different standing position or sit on the board in the **Clownfish Get Set** position (Fig. 8-38).

3. Use eight **Cruise Forward** arm strokes while in **Stand Up** position; then, **Bend Up** and grasp the ends of the board. Push board straight down and extend legs to the back (Fig. 8-78). Flutter or breast stroke kick forward 16 times. Return to the **Stand Up** position and repeat the sequence across the pool.

NOTE: Also combine movements from any two groups of Aquabatics. For example, pull yourself across the pool in **Stretch**

Long on Back from the **Flounder**; return in **Knees Up** position from the **Clownfish**.

IDEAS COMBINING VIGOROUS ARM AND LEG MOVEMENTS FROM "KICKBOARDING," "AQUABATICS," AND "WALK, JOG, JUMP, HOP, AND KICK" SECTIONS

1. Use **Water Boatman** or **Surfbird** kicks from the "Kickboarding" section. Travel across the pool using one style of kick; return using another.
2. Walk, jog, jump, or hop across the pool using movements from the **Snail, Lily Trotter, Dolphin,** or **Sand Hopper** groups (from the "Walk, Jog, Jump, Hop, and Kick" chapter). Move across using one style; return using another. As you move along, push the board on the surface in front, pull it from behind, or hold it on top of your head or overhead.
3. Move across the pool using any movement under #1 above; return using any movement under #2.
4. During #1, #2, or #3 above, stop in the center of the pool and do brisk movements in place from the **Dolphin** or **Sand Hopper** groups or arm movements from **Crocodile** Aquabatics (p. 150).
5. During #1, #2, or #3 above, stop at the opposite side of the pool, set the board on the ledge and hold the pool rim. Then, kick or jump using Aquacises from **Salmon** (p. 93) or **Bounce on the Wall** (p. 86), from the "Walk, Jog, Jump, Hop, and Kick" chapter.
6. Move across the pool using your legs as in #1 or #2 above. To return, pull with your arms while perched atop the board in positions from **Clownfish, Flounder, Swan,** or **Flamingo** Aquabatics.

MISCELLANEOUS IDEAS FOR TRAVELING ACROSS THE POOL IN WAIST-TO-CHEST-DEEP WATER

1. Move across two widths of the pool with a partner. Partners should face each other holding one board between them at the surface, hands holding onto each end (Fig. 8-100). Then, they should walk quickly sideways to the center and step around to change places (keeping hands in place on the board) before continuing across. Take huge steps and bring feet together with each one. To return, one partner walks forward while the other walks backward. Exchange places again in the center and continue to the starting point. Or, instead of changing places, stop and swing the board in large circles, pushing it beneath the surface, then swinging it overhead. Circle several times in each direction.

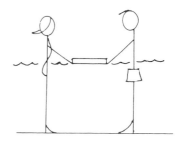

FIGURE 8-100

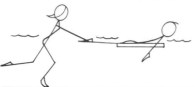

FIGURE 8-101

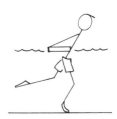

FIGURE 8-102

2. Move across two widths of the pool with a partner. Partner #1 should lie with the board lengthwise under his stomach while Partner #2 stands behind, holding the other's feet. Partner #2 then runs forward pushing #1 ahead (Fig. 8-101). Partner #2 can substitute a flutter or breast stroke kick while #1 pulls with his arms. Exchange places for the return trip. Three hints: (1) Place board so the lower end extends past hip joints to keep legs close to the surface. (2) Legs of Partner #1 should be kept straight. (3) Partner #2 should push with straight elbows.

3. Hop across the pool with one leg elevated, toes curled over the straight end of the board (Fig. 8-102). Change to the other leg in the center and continue across. To return, run forward while holding the board behind at the surface. Hold it crosswise, arms on top, fingers gripping the outside edges (Fig. 8-103).

4. Move across the pool using your legs as in **Pedal** (Fig. 8-71). To return, turn around to face the starting point, then (a) sit on the board and pull with your arms or (b) sit down in the water and guide the board across with your chin resting on the straight end (Fig. 8-104). Use arms as explained on p. 27. Pull smoothly to avoid turbulence, or (c) hop across on one foot with board locked behind the other knee (Fig. 8-105). Use arms to help pull you along.

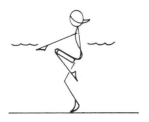

FIGURE 8-103

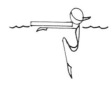

FIGURE 8-104

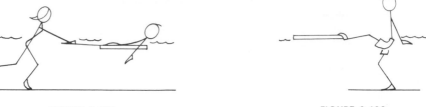

FIGURE 8-105

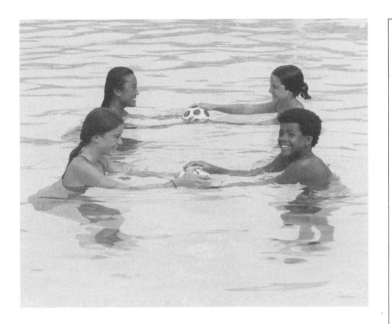

Have a (Beach) Ball!

Beach Ball Aquacises are simply what their name implies—eleven diverse groups of movements using a beach ball and ranging in difficulty from easy to hard. Most people who can float on their front and back and recover to a standing position can do them, although the **Diatom** and **Pink Fairy** groups require some swimming proficiency because they take place in deeper water. In addition, **Squid** and some movements in "More Beach Ball Ideas" call for the use of the flutter or breast stroke kick.

Some movements, such as **Shoveler** and **Mussel**, primarily firm and tone muscles of the arms and upper trunk, while **Balloon Fish** is designed for the thighs and lower trunk. **Sea Moth** and **Anchovy** stretch and firm your midsection and shoulders, while **Sunfish** stretches your legs and tests your balance. **Stinker, Capybara,** and **Diatom** test your balance; firm your inner thighs, arms, and trunk; and increase flexibility of the spine as well. However, expect some initial soreness in your inner thighs from gripping the ball tightly with your knees. **Pink Fairy** is the ultimate test of your balance and coordination and, finally, **Ballyhoo** (super for legs and feet), **Squid,** and "More Beach Ball Ideas" further increase your cardiovascular fitness.

Selected Beach Ball Aquacises can be used as part of your fitness session or use them as the basis for an entire program as explained in "Water Workouts Program C." Some

Beach Ball Aquacises

SHOVELER (p. 173)
  Shove Down
  Shove Down—Push Front
  Shove Down—Push Side
  Shove Down—Up
  Shove Down—Tuck and Touch
  Shove 'n Circle
  Shove Down—Turn and Catch
  Shove Side—Back—Side
  Knee Up—Shove Under
  Shove Down—Shove Out
  Shove Down—Swing Across
  Shove Down—Circle Around
MUSSEL (p. 176)
  Basic Movement
ANCHOVY (p. 176)
  Basic Movement
SEA MOTH (p. 177)
  Pull Down—Press Up
  Bend Side—Tuck-In
  Twist—Tuck-In
  Bend Forward—Bend Back
  Stretch Diagonal
  Push Away—Pull Back
  Halo
BALLOON FISH (p. 178)
  Kick Up—Kick Back
  Surface Arc
  Push Down—Kick Side
  Push Down—Kick Across
SUNFISH (p. 180)
  Levitate Legs Back
  Levitate to Slant—Roll Over
  Levitate to Vertical, Legs V-Split
  Levitate, V-Split Legs Back
  Levitate V-Split 'n Sit
  Take Turns
  Touch 'n Stand
  Touch, Lift, Press Down 'n Stand
  Touch 'n Lift
  Tootsie

STINKER (p. 182)
  Tuck to Vertical
  Tuck to Semi-Arch
  Tuck to Arch
  Tuck Right—Tuck Left
  Tuck 'n Circle
  Vertical to Arch
  Horizontal Swing
  Vertical to Pike
  Pike to Arch
  Oscillate
CAPYBARA (p. 185)
  Float 'n Tuck to Vertical
  Float 'n Tuck to Semi-Arch
  Float 'n Tuck to Arch
  Arch and Pull
  Tuck and Pull
  Spin
  Applaud
  Double Arm and Knee Swing
  Circle Knees
  Float 'n Oscillate
DIATOM (p. 187)
  Hang Up
  Hang Up—Toes Up
  Cruise Forward or Backward
  Spin or Applaud
  Hang Up—Twist
  Hang Up—Arms Up and Down
  Hang UP—Bend Up
  Hang Up—Pike Up
  Pike and Pull
  Hang Up—Float Up
PINK FAIRY (p. 188)
  Basic Movement
  Cruise Forward, or Backward
  Spin, Applaud, or Twist
  Arms Up and Down
  Bend Up
  Bend Up and Pull
  The Creep
  One Foot Stand

resemble kickboard Aquabatics, but you will find that they will all challenge your balance and coordination in many new ways.

The size of the ball is important. It should be large enough to offer plenty of resistance (or support you in **Capybara, Diatom,** and **Pink Fairy**) yet small enough to push beneath the surface. Generally, a 25 to 29 inch circumference ball is suitable for all categories, although men may want to use a slightly larger one.

SHOVELER

Firms and strengthens hands, arms, and all muscles of the trunk

GET SET: Stand erect in **waist-to-chest-deep water** with your feet apart side to side and hold a 25 to 29 inch ball as instructed below. For best results, stabilize your body by pulling in your stomach and keeping your feet on the floor. If your feet leave the floor, either move to shallower water (not less than waist deep) or use a smaller ball.

GO: Choose a variety of Aquacises from this list and repeat each ten to twenty times. Or, combine several of them into a sequence by repeating each six times before moving to the next. For a balanced workout, use both forward and sideward movements, adding some backward ones from the **Sea Moth** (p. 177). During each **Shoveler** movement, shove the ball down forcefully, then let it rise slowly by resisting its upward pressure.

Shove Down. Start by holding the ball at the surface close to your chest. Now, shove the ball down until elbows are straight (Fig. 9-1), then bend elbows and let ball rise to the start. Keep back erect and elbows close to your body.

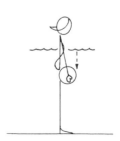

FIGURE 9-1

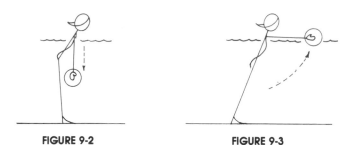

FIGURE 9-2   FIGURE 9-3   FIGURE 9-4

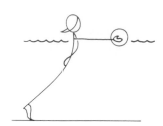

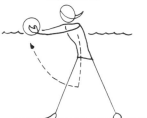

FIGURE 9-5

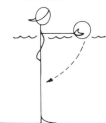

FIGURE 9-6

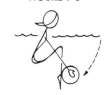

FIGURE 9-7

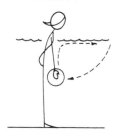

FIGURE 9-8

Shove Down—Push Front. Hold the ball at the surface close to your chest. Now, bend forward slightly, and shove the ball straight down as far as possible (Fig. 9-2). Then, move it slowly forward and up to the surface (Fig. 9-3). Reverse the motion by pulling ball down to your legs, then bend elbows and let it rise to the SP as you straighten up. Keep heels on the floor. To vary, let your weight fall forward and rise to your toes as the ball moves forward (Fig. 9-4). Hold briefly as you stretch legs, tighten buttocks, and lift chest; then press hips back and pull in your stomach hard as you pull ball down to your legs. Finally, bend elbows and stand erect, letting ball rise to the surface SP.

Shove Down—Push Side. Hold the ball at the surface close to your chest. Now, shove the ball straight down, then move it up to the surface at the side (Fig. 9-5). Reverse the motion by pushing ball down as you turn forward, then bend elbows and let ball rise slowly to the SP. Alternate sides. To vary, intersperse this movement with **Shove Down—Push Forward.**

Shove Down—Up. Start by holding the ball at the surface in front, elbows straight. Now, with elbows straight, shove the ball down toward your legs (Fig. 9-6), then reverse the motion by moving ball slowly forward to the SP.

Shove Down—Tuck and Touch. This time, stand in **chest-to-shoulder-deep water** and hold the ball forward on the surface. Now, lift knees at the same time you press ball down to touch it to the tops of your feet (Fig. 9-7). Reverse the motion to the SP. Keep elbows straight and feet together.

Shove 'n Circle. Start with the ball at the surface in front, elbows straight. Shove it down toward your legs, then bend elbows and let is rise almost to the surface. Push ball forward to the SP (Fig. 9-8) and repeat the circling motion several times before reversing direction. Always keep ball submerged.

Shove Down—Turn and Catch. Hold the ball on the surface close to your chest. Now, press ball down between your legs and then turn quickly to catch it as it pops up behind.

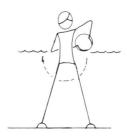

FIGURE 9-9

Shove Side—Back—Side. Place a 25 inch ball on the surface next to your left side and hold it with your right hand behind your back, left arm sideward, hand on top of the ball (Fig. 9-9). Now, press the ball down, skimming it along your left side, past your legs in back, then up your right side. Reverse the motion back to the start. Keep back erect and straighten elbows on the downward motion. If shoulder flexibility is limited at first, perform in **waist-deep water.** Or, begin by holding the ball with your right arm in *front* (Fig. 9-10). Then, skim it down your side, across in *front* of your legs, and up your right side.

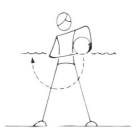

FIGURE 9-10

Knee Up—Shove Under. Hold a 25 inch ball at the surface on your right, right hand on top. Now, lift your right knee and press the ball under it (Fig. 9-11). Next, let ball rise in front, grasp it with your left hand, and swing it in a wide arc across the surface to the left. Lift left knee and press the ball under; let it rise in front again and use your right hand to move it in a wide arc around to the start.

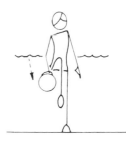

FIGURE 9-11

Shove Down—Shove Out. Hold the ball close to your side at the surface, hand on top. Now, press the ball down, sliding it along your side until elbow is straight; then push the ball sideward letting it rise slowly to the surface (Fig. 9-12). Reverse the motion by pressing ball down and toward you, keeping elbow straight. Finally, bend elbow and let ball rise slowly to the SP. If this reverse motion is too difficult at first, simply bend elbow and pull ball toward you along the surface to the SP. After several repetitions, do it with the opposite arm.

Shove Down—Swing Across. Hold a 25 inch ball out to one side at the surface, elbow straight. Next, press it down and across in front of your legs and up to the surface at the other side (Fig. 9-13). Reverse the action and return to the start.

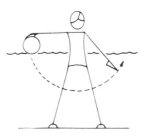

FIGURE 9-13

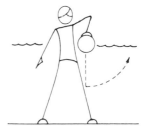

FIGURE 9-12

Repeat several times before changing to the opposite arm. To vary, (1) change ball to the other hand as you move it across in front or (2) move ball behind your legs and grasp it with the opposite hand as it passes across in back.

Shove Down—Circle Around. Hold a 25 inch ball close to your chest at the surface, right hand on top. Now, press ball straight down, then swing it in a wide circle around your body, changing to the left hand as it passes in back. Change again to the right hand as it moves across in front. Repeat several times, circling in the same direction, or change direction with each circle. Keep working arm straight. Periodically perform with the left arm.

You also can use a ball for the following "Shape-Ups":

Sawfish (p. 38). Keep ball just under the surface and swing it around, touching it to your waist at each side.

Trunkfish (p. 37). Use the ball for all **Trunkfish** movements but be careful to hold it extra tight on all downward movements. Keep ball always under the surface.

Hydra. Variation, **Circle in Unison,** (p. 32).

MUSSEL

Firms and strengthens muscles of arms and chest

GET SET: Stand in **waist-deep water** with your feet apart side to side. Hold the ball between your hands in front at shoulder level, arms straight.

GO: Press both hands against the ball. At the same time, slowly rotate the ball left and then right, maintaining constant pressure on the ball (Fig. 9-14). Rotate three times in each direction and gradually increase to 10. You also may hold the ball just beneath the surface as you rotate it.

ANCHOVY

Tones arms and trunk; increases flexibility of spine and shoulders

GET SET: Start by floating on your back, feet together, and hold the ball on the surface (Fig. 9-15). Tuck-in and stretch legs.

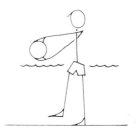

FIGURE 9-14

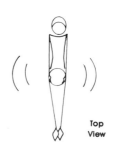

Top
View

FIGURE 9-15

GO: Swing the ball to the right along the surface to a position overhead as you roll to your right side (Fig. 9-16). Stretch briefly, pressing heels back, legs just under the surface; then reverse the motion to the left, rolling to your left side. Keep legs and arms straight, feet extended and together. Swing the ball with gusto and, for greater challenges, swing it half submerged or just under the surface. Start with 6 repetitions to each side and work up to 15. For further variety, try **Whirlabout** (p. 163), using a ball instead of a kickboard.

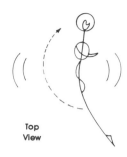

Top
View

FIGURE 9-16

SEA MOTH

Trims and firms midsection; increases flexibility of trunk, chest, and shoulders

GET SET: Stand in **waist-to-chest-deep water** with feet apart side to side and hold the ball as instructed below. Pull in your stomach.

GO: Choose your favorites from this group and repeat each 8 to 15 times. Better yet, do several of them in sequence, repeating each six times before moving to the next. Keep shoulders down and relaxed. And, whenever the ball is overhead, press elbows back to stretch chest and shoulders to improve posture.

Pull Down—Press Up. Stand erect and Tuck-in. Hold the ball overhead and back as far as possible, elbows straight. Now, bend elbows and lower ball *straight down* in back without touching the back of your head or moving your head forward. Then, press it straight up to the start, keeping elbows pressed back at all times.

Bend Side—Tuck-In. Stretch up, holding the ball overhead with elbows straight. Hold the stretch and bend from side to side, tucking-in each time you straighten up. To vary, after bending once to each side, either: (1) Bend your elbows and touch the ball to your chest. Lift ball overhead and repeat the sequence. (2) Bend elbows and lower ball behind head as described in **Pull Down—Press Up.** Lift ball overhead and repeat. (3) Alternate (1) with (2). (4) Bend elbows and lower the ball to chest level, then toss it straight up and catch it. Straighten arms overhead and repeat the sequence.

Twist—Tuck-In. Hold the ball overhead with elbows straight and stretch upward. Hold the stretch as you twist to the right from the waist and press your right elbow back (Fig. 9-17); twist

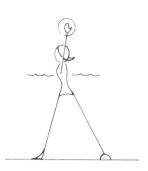

FIGURE 9-17

forward and Tuck-in. Repeat to the left. To vary: (1) Perform with feet far apart and hold the ball against the back of your neck. Keep head erect, elbows pressed back, and heels on the floor. Or, (2) after twisting once to each side, use any **Bend Side— Tuck In** variation.

Bend Forward—Bend Back. Stand with feet far apart. Bend forward from the hips and hold the ball just above the surface in front, elbows straight. Tuck-in, pressing hips back and stretching arms forward (Fig. 9-18). Now, lift the ball overhead, stretching up and back as you push hips forward, tighten buttocks, and lift your chest (Fig. 9-19). Move smoothly from one position to the other, holding each for several seconds (but avoid holding your breath).

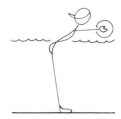

FIGURE 9-18

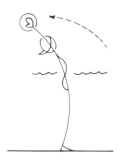

Stretch Diagonal. Do **Bend Forward—Bend Backward,** but instead of bending directly forward, bend diagonally forward— first to the right (Fig. 9-20); swing the ball overhead, then bend diagonally forward to the left. Lower ball nearly to the water's surface each time.

FIGURE 9-19

Push Away—Pull Back. Use **Bend Forward—Bend Back** SP and movement but this time pull the ball back to your chest (Fig. 9-21) instead of lifting it overhead.

Halo.

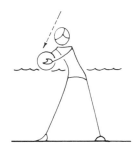

1. Swing the ball overhead in large circles by combining **Bend Forward—Bend Back** and **Bend Side** movements. Begin with the ball forward just above the surface, hips pressed back. Now, swing ball sideward, around to the back, over to the other side, then forward to the start. Move slowly, stopping to stretch momentarily in each of the four positions. Or, circle in a continuous, sweeping motion. Periodically change direction.

FIGURE 9-20

2. Swing ball briskly in smaller circles. Keep legs stiff, heels on the floor, and arms locked into position with the ball directly overhead. Pull in your stomach and feel the action strongly in your midsection. To vary, perform several sequences alternating four repetitions each of versions #1 and #2.

BALLOON FISH

Improves balance and coordination; tones muscles of lower trunk and thighs

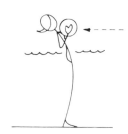

GET SET: Stand with feet together in **waist-to-chest-deep water** and hold the ball as instructed below. Pull in your stomach.

FIGURE 9-21

GO: Choose your favorites and repeat each 15 to 25 times; or, do them all in sequence, repeating each four to six times before moving to the next. Be sure to perform an equal number of repetitions with the opposite leg.

Kick Up—Kick Back. Hold the ball in front at the surface, elbows straight, and bend forward from the hips. Now, keeping the ball in position, kick one leg up to the front, then down and up to the back, knee straight (Fig. 9-22). Try to lift toes to the ball in front and your heel to the surface in back.

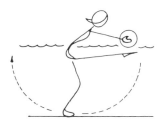

FIGURE 9-22

Surface Arc. Hold the ball in front at the surface, elbows straight, and lift your right leg to the back (Fig. 9-23). Now swing the ball across the surface to the right as you swing your leg in an arc to the front, keeping toes close to the surface (Fig. 9-24). Reverse the motion back to the start. Keep elbows and working knee straight and press down on the ball as you swing it. Stretch to your maximum by swinging arms and leg as far as possible in each direction to get the most waist exercise.

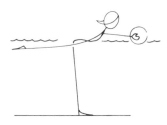

FIGURE 9-23

Push Down—Kick Side. Hold the ball close to your chest at the surface. Now, push it straight down as you kick one leg to the side, foot flexed (Fig. 9-25). Reverse the action and return to the start; then repeat, alternating legs. Keep working knee straight but, if desired, bend your supporting knee as you kick up, then straighten it as you return to the start.

Push Down—Kick Across. Stand erect holding the ball at the right, elbows bent (Fig. 9-26). Now, kick your right leg diagonally across in front as you press the ball straight down (Fig. 9-27). Return to the start, then swing ball around to the left side and repeat with the left leg. Keep working knee straight but, if desired, bend supporting knee as you kick up.

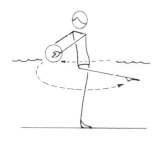

FIGURE 9-24

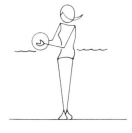

FIGURE 9-26

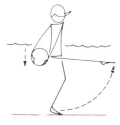

FIGURE 9-27

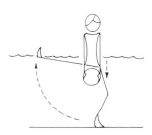

FIGURE 9-25

SUNFISH

Increases strength and flexibility of trunk muscles; strengthens arms and hands; improves coordination

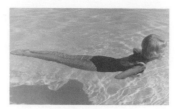

FIGURE 9-28

GET SET: Stand in **chest-deep water** holding the ball as suggested in each of the following Aquacises.

GO: Use the first movement until balance and coordination improve, then move one by one through the entire group until you have mastered them all. Change position slowly, always stretching to your limit.

Levitate Legs Back. Stand with feet together and hold the ball against your midsection, elbows pointing to the side. Now, lean forward and let your straight legs rise to the surface in back (Fig. 9-28). Balance in this position for a count of eight while you lift chin and heels, tighten buttocks, and stretch. To return to the upright SP, first tuck knees toward chest, then lower feet to the floor. To aid balance while floating, separate legs to a wide V-split if desired. Bring legs together before returning to the SP. Start with 6 and work up to 12 repetitions. To vary, open legs to V, then close them several times while in floating position.

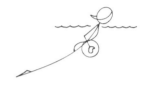

FIGURE 9-29

Levitate to Slant—Roll Over. Hold ball as suggested in the first movement, then lean forward and let legs rise in back only until body is on a slant (Fig. 9-29). Now, roll onto your back, slightly bending legs forward at the hip (Fig. 9-30). Hold briefly, then continue to roll in the same direction to the SP. Do several revolutions in each direction or change direction after each.

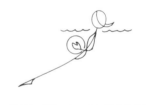

FIGURE 9-30

Remember: (1) Avoid turning your head—keep it in line with your body. (2) Hold legs together, feet extended. (3) Tighten muscles of buttocks, stomach, and legs. (4) A slight rotation of the hips is all that is needed to initiate the rolling action. You also can roll by moving the ball slightly to the right or left (keeping ball in contact with midsection). (5) Placement of the ball is important—if it is placed too high, you move into a vertical position; if it is placed too low, your legs will rise too high.

Levitate to Vertical, Legs V-Split. Stand on tiptoe with feet apart and hold the ball close to your chest at the surface. Now, press the ball straight down in front, then separate legs even farther so that you are floating with feet off the pool floor (Fig. 9-31). Balance in this position for a slow count of eight with back erect, arms close to body, and elbows straight. Tuck-in

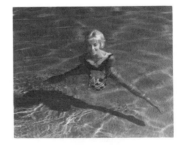

FIGURE 9-31

and stretch legs, feet extended. Bring toes to the floor and bend elbows, letting ball rise slowly to the surface while you resist its upward pressure. Keep legs separated the entire time.

Levitate, V-Split Legs Back. Stand on tiptoe with feet apart and hold the ball close to your chest at the surface. Push the ball straight down. Now, lean forward and let your straight legs rise to the surface in back. Hold the extended position with heels and chin lifted, buttocks and leg muscles taut (Fig. 9-32). Next, push legs down to the feet-apart SP by exhaling and pulling in stomach tightly. Stand upright, then bend elbows and let ball rise to the surface SP. Start with 6 and work up to 12 repetitions. To vary, lower and raise legs several times from the floating position, then stand. Keep legs straight and always in a wide V-split.

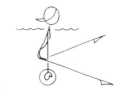

FIGURE 9-32

Levitate V-Split 'n Sit. Start by holding the ball and standing on tiptoe as suggested above. Push the ball straight down. This time, lift legs forward to a high, wide V-split on either side of your arms (Fig. 9-33). Push legs down to the SP, keeping knees straight and legs separated to the maximum. To vary, begin and end each up-down leg movement standing on your heels (Fig. 9-34). Perform briskly, keeping knees straight and feet flexed.

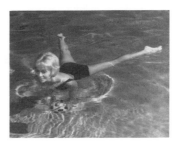

FIGURE 9-33

Take Turns. Alternate between **V-Split Legs Back** and **V-Split 'n Sit,** as previously described, bringing toes to the floor after each up-down leg motion. Keep legs separated and stretched to the maximum. Perform either with ball pressed straight down the entire time or bend elbows and let ball rise slowly to the surface between each up-down leg motion. Start with 8 complete movements and work up to 15.

Touch 'n Stand. Stand on tiptoe, feet apart side to side, and hold the ball straight down in front (Fig. 9-35). Now, bend your knees outward and lift heels to sides of ball (Fig. 9-36); then straighten knees, bringing feet down to the SP. Repeat 8 times and increase to 20.

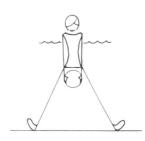

FIGURE 9-34

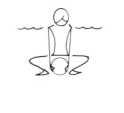

FIGURE 9-36

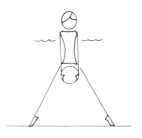

FIGURE 9-35

Touch, Lift, Press Down, 'n Stand. Touch heels to the ball as in the movement above, then straighten knees, lifting legs to a high, wide V-split with feet flexed (Fig. 9-37). Press legs down, extending feet and ending in the tiptoe SP. To vary, begin and end this movement standing on your heels (Fig. 9-34). Keeping feet flexed, touch and lift as instructed, then touch heels to ball again before standing. Start with 8 repetitions and work up to 20. For these and the following movements, to avoid tipping over backward as legs move up, incline trunk forward slightly and hold ball straight down.

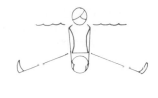

FIGURE 9-37

Touch 'n Lift. Omit returning feet to the floor each time. Instead, alternately touch heels to the ball, then straighten legs to a high V-split. Repeat the knee bending-straightening action 10 times and work up to 20. Try to lift toes to the surface and keep legs separated as far as possible.

Tootsie. Hold the ball straight down and balance with legs in a high V-split while alternately flexing and extending your feet 10 to 20 times.

Note. Swimmers also can do **Sunfish** Aquacises in deep water where their feet cannot touch the floor.

STINKER

Firms and strengthens muscles of inner thighs, waist, abdomen, lower back, and buttocks. Holding pool rim strengthens hands, arms, and upper body

GET SET: With a 25 inch ball pressed firmly between your knees, face the wall in **chest-deep water** and hold the pool rim with hands shoulder-width apart. However, this spacing may increase depending on the size ball, so position hands for greatest leverage.

GO: Starting with **Tuck to Vertical,** gain control of each movement before moving to the next one. Concentrate on pressing your knees tightly against the ball and lift them forward only as far as needed to maintain control. Otherwise, this exercise can truly be a "stinker" because lifting the knees high makes it easier for the ball to pop loose and surprise you with a "clop in the chops." This possibility increases as the inner thigh muscles tire, so do only a few repetitions at first. However, as your thighs strengthen, you'll soon be able to control the ball and increase the lift.

Tuck to Vertical. Start with knees tucked up in front, legs close to the wall as in Fig. 9-38. Now, alternately press knees down until thighs are vertical (Fig. 9-39), then lift knees up to the start. In the beginning, you can raise knees only halfway to the surface but, as you gain control over the ball, strive to bring them up to the surface. Start with 4 and work up to 20 repetitions. Keep stomach pulled in, back erect, and upper body still.

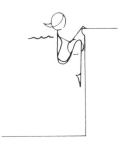

FIGURE 9-38

Tuck to Semi-Arch. Perform **Tuck to Vertical,** but this time press your knees down and back to the semi-arch position shown in Fig. 9-40. Hold the arch briefly with head erect, chest lifted, and buttocks tight, then pull in your stomach even more as you tuck knees up to the start. Repeat 4 times and work up to 20. Inhale as you arch; exhale as you tuck up.

Tuck to Arch. Start again with knees tucked up in front. Now, lean forward and press your knees down, then up to the surface in back (Fig. 9-41). You can brace your elbows against the wall for leverage as knees move down, but they should straighten as legs move up to the back. Briefly stretch in the arched position as you lift your feet and tighten your buttocks; then pull in your stomach hard and, in one smooth motion, forcefully push knees down and forward to the SP. Repeat 4 times and gradually increase to 20.

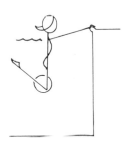

FIGURE 9-39

Tuck Right—Tuck Left. Start in the arched position shown in Fig. 9-41 (with elbows straight). Now, swing your knees around to your right elbow, bending the left elbow to brace it against the wall for leverage. Reverse the motion by swinging knees back

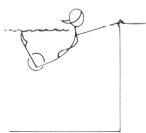

FIGURE 9-40

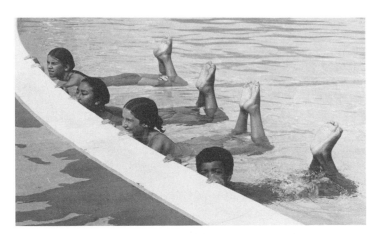

FIGURE 9-41

past the start and toward your left elbow as you brace your right elbow. Swing knees from side to side in this manner, keeping stomach pulled in and ball gripped firmly between knees. Start with 4 and work up to 15 repetitions to each side.

Tuck 'n Circle. Starting in the arched position (Fig. 9-41), tuck knees to your right elbow as instructed above. However, this time continue the circular motion by swinging knees across in front to your left elbow, then around to the back SP. Start with 4 circles in each direction and gradually increase to 15. To vary, alternate the direction of each circle.

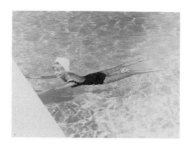

Vertical to Arch. Stand on the floor, arms' length from the wall, holding the ledge with elbows straight and with the ball gripped between knees. Now, lean forward, letting legs rise to the surface in back (Fig. 9-42). Hold this position and stretch for a slow count of eight with buttocks tight and heels and chin lifted. Next, pull in your stomach and forcefully press legs down to the start, keeping knees straight the entire time. Start with 4, increase to 10.

FIGURE 9-42

Horizontal Swing. From the position shown in Fig. 9-42, perform the movement described in **Surface Fishtail** (p. 45). Keep leg and buttocks muscles taut, heels lifted. Start with 6 in each direction and work up to 15.

Vertical to Pike. Stand on the floor, arms' length from the wall, and hold the ledge with hands shoulder-width apart, arms straight and ball between knees. Now, let legs rise forward to a pike position with knees straight, feet flat on the wall (Fig. 9-43); then press legs down to the start. Concentrate on gripping the ball firmly. Start with 6 repetitions and work up to 15.

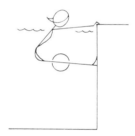

Pike to Arch. Move smoothly between the arch and pike positions shown in Figs. 9-42 and 9-43. Hold each position briefly, keeping your stomach pulled in and the ball gripped firmly between your straight knees. Feet do not touch the floor as legs swing past vertical. Start with 6 and work up to 15 repetitions.

FIGURE 9-43

Oscillate. For this final movement in the **Stinker** group, roll onto your back and hold the pool rim with arms sideward and straight. Either brace the back of your head against the wall or rest the back of your neck on the rim. Hold the ball firmly between your knees (Fig. 9-44). Now, briskly swing knees from side to side, twisting at the waist and pushing knees down into the water at each side. As you roll from one hip to the other, keep shoulders level and stomach pulled in. **Oscillate** 8 times to each side and gradually increase to 15.

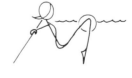

FIGURE 9-44

CAPYBARA

Strengthens and firms muscles of inner thighs and trunk; arm movements add arm and upper body exercise

GET SET: Swimmers, for these follow-ons to **Stinker** movements, move away from the wall into **chest-deep water** with a 25 inch ball gripped firmly between your knees.

FIGURE 9-45

GO: Start this group of Aquacises using the first movement and get the knack of each one before progressing to the next. Always keep hands under the surface.

Float 'n Tuck to Vertical. With arms forward at the surface, palms down, alternately tuck up knees (Fig. 9-45) then push them down until thighs are vertical (Fig. 9-46). Keep arm motion to a minimum and rely on trunk and thigh muscles to provide the needed control. At first, lift knees forward only halfway, then after inner thigh muscles are stronger, lift knees up to your elbows. Start with 8 repetitions and work up to 20.

Float 'n Tuck to Semi-Arch. From the position shown in Fig. 9-45, press knees down and back to a semi-arch position (Fig. 9-47). At the same time, move arms out to the side and back just under the surface. Hold the arch briefly as you tighten buttocks and lift chest. (If necessary for balance, paddle gently with hands.) Then, pull in stomach hard and move arms and knees forward to the SP. Start with 8 and work up to 20 repetitions. To vary, on the forward motion, clasp arms around knees.

FIGURE 9-46

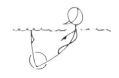

Float 'n Tuck to Arch. From the position shown in Fig. 9-45, press knees and arms back until you tip forward onto your stomach and your feet emerge in back. Next, to prepare for return to the SP, slide arms forward then briefly stretch in the arched position (Fig. 9-48). Return to the start by forcefully pressing arms down as you lift knees forward. Start with 6 and work up to 15 repetitions.

FIGURE 9-47

Arch and Pull. Perform the above movement and, during the arch portion, quickly stroke across the pool pulling arms as in dog paddle, freestyle, or as used in **Cruise Headfirst** (p. 161). To return to the SP in Fig. 9-45, press arms down and lift knees forward.

Tuck and Pull. Using arms **Oarfish** style (p. 27), move back and forth across the pool with knees facing up (Fig. 9-45), forward (Fig. 9-49), and down (Fig. 9-46). Repeat several sequences of eight strokes with knees in each position. For *variety*, repeat several sequences of eight strokes with body arched (Fig. 9-48), alternated with eight, knees tucked up (Fig. 9-45).

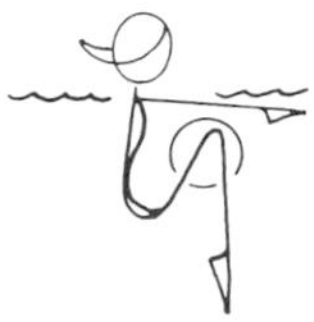

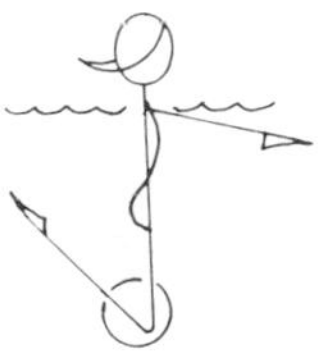

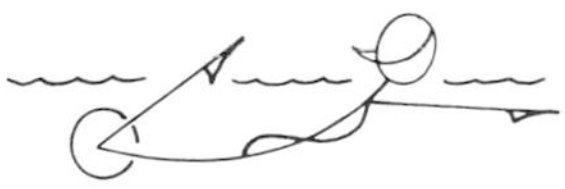

FIGURE 9-48

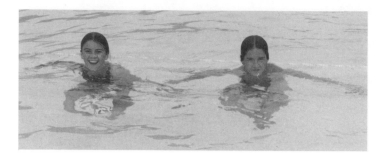

FIGURE 9-49

Spin. With back erect, turn in a circle with knees in each of the above positions. You can either pull one arm toward you, then immediately press outward with the other arm (hands just under the surface), or keep one hand on your hip while pulling inward with the other arm. Periodically change to the opposite arm and turn in the opposite direction. See how far you can turn on each forceful pull.

Applaud. With knees in each of the positions shown in Figs. 9-46 and 9-49, clap hands alternately in front and in back, under the surface. Turn palms to face the direction of movement and bring them together both in front and in back. Do 8 complete movements to start and work up to 15.

Double Arm and Knee Swing. With legs in each of the three positions shown in Figs. 9-45, 9-46, and 9-49, swing arms and knees from side to side, moving arms opposite to the direction of knees. Feel the twisting action in your waist. Start with arms out to each side, then move the left arm across in front as you move the right arm back. Reverse the motion, swinging arms around to the left. Swing smoothly and continuously, keeping hands close to the surface, palms tilted in the direction of movement. Begin with 4 swings to each side with knees in each of the 3 positions and work up to 8.

Circle Knees. Start with thighs vertical (Fig. 9-46) and with arms out to each side, hands at the surface. Now swing knees up to your right elbow, across in front to the left elbow, then down to the start. Repeat 6 times in each direction and work up to 15, or alternate the direction of each circle. Keep stomach pulled in, back erect, and knees pressed tightly against the ball.

Float 'n Oscillate. Perform **Oscillate** (p. 184) with body floating horizontally, head resting on the water, arms sideward at the surface (Fig. 9-50). Do 8 to each side and work up to 15.

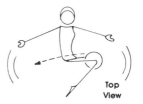

FIGURE 9-50

DIATOM

Tones and firms entire body

GET SET: Swimmers, suspend yourself vertically in at least **shoulder-deep water,** with a 25 inch ball pressed between your straight knees (Fig. 9-51).

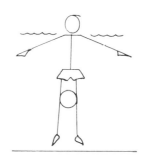

FIGURE 9-51

GO: Practice **Stinker** and **Capybara** before trying these movements, then do them one by one, gaining control over each before moving to the next. Always keep hands under the surface.

Hang Up. With arms sideward, hands at the surface, balance motionless in the **Get Set** position described above. Tuck-in tightly with back erect and legs stretched to keep muscles taut. At first, during this and the next movement, you can use gentle paddling or sculling hand movements to increase balance.

Hang Up—Toes Up. From the **Hang Up** position, alternately flex feet to point toes up, then extend them to point toes down. Keep legs stretched and muscles taut. Flex and extend 10 times and work up to 20.

Cruise Forward or Backward. For this movement, use arms as in **Oarfish** (p. 27).

Spin or **Applaud.** While in **Hang Up** position, use arms as described under those headings in the **Capybara** group (p. 186).

Hang Up—Twist. From **Hang Up** position, turn hips from side to side while gently swinging arms opposite to the direction of your hips as described in **Double Arm and Knee Swing** (p. 186). Start with 10 twists to each side and work up to 20.

Hang Up—Arms Up and Down. From **Hang Up,** bounce up and down in the water by using arms **Butterflyfish** style (p. 26). If you like, completely submerge each time by pushing arms with extra force. Keep body in straight alignment and pull arms evenly. Begin with 8 down-up arm motions and increase to 20.

Hang Up—Bend Up. From **Hang Up** position, hold arms forward at the surface, palms down. Alternately tuck up your knees then extend legs down to the start. Try to lift knees to elbows. Repeat 10 to 20 times.

Hang Up—Pike Up. Start in **Hang Up** position, arms sideward, hands just under the surface. Now, pike legs forward as you scoop arms forward to touch fingers to toes (Fig. 9-52). Press legs down and pull arms back to the SP. Move slowly from one position to the other, keeping hands just under the surface, stomach in, legs stretched and tensed. Repeat 8 times and work up to 20.

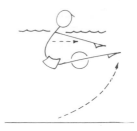

FIGURE 9-52

Pike and Pull. From **Pike Up** position (Fig. 9-52), pull yourself forward through the water using arms in a simulated breast stroke as in **Oarfish** (p. 27). Keep back erect and legs stretched forward at right angles to body. Also use the reverse arm motion to sail backward. Move forward one pool width then move backward one width, or do several sequences of eight forward strokes alternating with eight backward ones.

Hang Up—Float Up. Starting in the **Hang Up** position, lean forward, letting legs rise to the surface in back as you move arms forward to a wide V (Fig. 9-53). To return to the SP, press arms down and bend knees toward chest to bring your trunk upright, then extend legs straight down. Concentrate on pressing knees constantly against the ball to keep it in place. This is a difficult manuever and may require a slightly smaller ball at first. Also, perform in shallower **waist-to-chest deep water** for greater ease. Start with 4 and work up to 10.

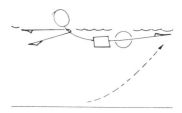

FIGURE 9-53

PINK FAIRY

Tones body, firms arms, and develops balance
and coordination

Swimmers! When you can do **Stinker, Capybara,** and **Diatom** Aquacises, try these—the ultimate challenges to your balance and coordination.

GET SET: Start in *calm* water deep enough to permit you to stand on a 25 inch ball without it touching the pool floor. To get into position, first suspend yourself as shown in Fig. 9-31. Then,

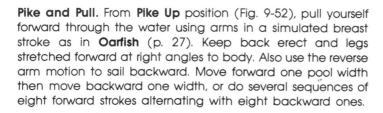

with arms vertical and ball pressed straight down, lift knees and curl soles of feet around sides of ball. (Keep face above the surface and tip head forward just enough to watch this action.) Next, release hands and straighten body and legs to vertical (Fig. 9-54). If you start to fall over, bend knees up and grasp ball to keep it from rocketing into an unwary swimmer. Then—try again!

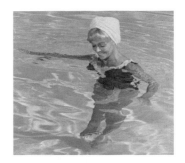

FIGURE 9-54

GO: Balance in the **Get Set** position with stomach pulled in, legs and buttocks taut. You can paddle hands gently under the surface; however, the idea is to keep arm motion to a minimum and rely on straight body alignment to stay upright. Now, you're ready to try the following movements:

Cruise Forward or Backward. Do this movement while standing on the ball and pulling arms **Oarfish** style (p. 27).

Spin, Applaud or **Twist.** Use your arms as described under **Spin** and **Applaud** (p. 186). To twist, swing arms as described on p. 186 under the heading of **Double Arm and Knee Swing.**

Arms Up and Down. Keeping feet in position, bounce up and down by using arms as described in **Butterflyfish** (p. 26). Pull arms evenly and keep body straight from head to foot. Do 8 to 12 repetitions.

FIGURE 9-55

Bend Up. Balance on the ball and hold arms forward, slightly more than shoulder-width apart, with hands at the surface, palms down. Now, alternately bend and straighten your knees. Move slowly with control and see if you can lift your knees up to your elbows. Start with 10, work up to 20 repetitions. To vary, balance for several seconds at a time with knees up (Fig. 9-55).

Bend Up and Pull. Cruise Forward or **Backward** while knees are bent, using arms **Oarfish** style (p. 27). Stroke forward one width of the pool, then backward one width, or repeat several sequences of eight forward strokes alternating with eight backward ones.

The Creep. Slowly slide feet together so that you're standing on top of the ball (Fig. 9-56). Then you can gently pull yourself forward and backward through the water.

One Foot Stand. Climax your stunning balancing act by standing with only one foot on top of the ball. With some practice, you can do it!

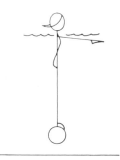

FIGURE 9-56

BALLYHOO

Develops endurance while strengthening muscles of feet, legs, and trunk

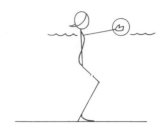

This group of jumping and hopping movements begins with the easier ones (holding the ball in your hands) and progresses to the harder movements (holding the ball between your knees).

FIGURE 9-57

GET SET: Start at one side of the pool in **waist-to-chest-deep** water in order to move back and forth across the pool.

GO: Use these movements singly for several widths of the pool. Or, to keep the action interesting and continuous, use a sequence of several by changing to a different movement for each width or two.

Jump on a Slant. Hold a 25 to 29 inch ball either on top of your head with elbows pressed back or on the surface in front, arms straight. Pull in your stomach. Now, lean forward from the ankles with your body straight and on a slant and jump up and down across the pool. (Holding the ball in front allows you to lean more.) Keep legs straight and use lots of foot action to push off vigorously. Land first on toes, then roll down to heels. On the up motion, tighten buttocks, stretch legs, and extend feet. The idea is to see how far you can lean without falling over.

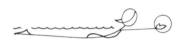

FIGURE 9-58

Run Forward on a Slant. This time, run forward with your body on a slant. Keep knees together and take tiny, fast steps on your toes. Hold the ball either on top of your head or against the back of your neck (in each case, keep head erect, elbows pressed back).

Run Backward on a Slant. Run backward with your body straight and slanted back, knees together. Hold the ball either (1) under your buttocks, (2) pressed against the lower back, (3) forward on the surface, (4) on top of your head, or (5) against the back of your neck. (Keep head erect and elbows pressed back.)

Push Off—Glide Forward. Start in **chest-deep water,** holding the ball on the surface in front. Bend knees to bring the water level over your shoulders (Fig. 9-57). Now, thrust yourself forward by vigorously pushing off the floor and lifting legs up to the back (Fig. 9-58). Glide briefly while you stretch legs, pull in stomach, and lift heels. Then, tuck up your knees (Fig. 9-59), lower feet to the floor, and immediately repeat, "surging" across the pool. To vary, (1) quickly open legs sideward to V-

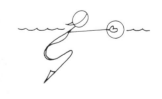

FIGURE 9-59

split, then close them while in the extended position and/or (2) as you tuck knees up, pull the ball toward you, pressing it several inches below the surface, then briefly touch ball to knees (Fig. 9-60). Immediately lower feet to the floor and extend arms forward to the SP before repeating the Aquacise.

Push Off—Glide Side. Stand with feet together and hold the ball on the surface at the left. Now, thrust yourself to the left by vigorously pushing your toes against the floor and lifting legs sideward (Fig. 9-61). Glide briefly with buttocks tight and legs stretched; then draw up knees until feet are under body. Place feet on the floor and stand. Repeat several times to the left, swing ball around to the right, and repeat to the right. Or, alternate from side to side. Keep legs together.

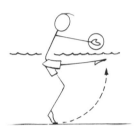

FIGURE 9-60

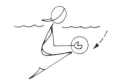

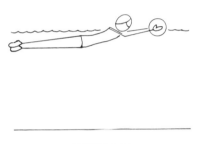

FIGURE 9-61

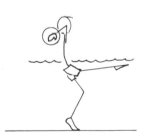

FIGURE 9-62

One Foot Hop with Ball in Front. Hold the ball on the surface in front, arms straight. Extend one leg forward, knee straight, toes at the surface (Fig. 9-62). Hop forward across the pool, keeping leg high and ball close to toes. Reverse legs for the return trip.

One Foot Hop with Ball High. Hop across the pool holding the ball behind your neck or atop your head and with one leg elevated as suggested below. Keep head and back erect, elbows pressed back. Try any or all of the following:

1. Hop forward or backward on one foot while lifting the other leg high in front—knee straight, toes at the surface (Fig. 9-63).
2. Hop forward or backward on one foot with the other leg extended back (Fig. 9-64).
3. Take four hops forward with the right leg forward. Then, keeping leg elevated, hop once turning left 180° by rotating at the hip joint. The right leg will then be extended back, putting you in position to hop four times backward. Hop/turn forward again and continue the sequence across the pool.

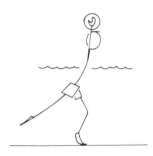

FIGURE 9-63

FIGURE 9-64

During all three versions, as well as those that follow, thrust yourself upward vigorously, momentarily straightening your supporting knee and extending your foot. Then, bend that knee as you land on the ball of your foot. Periodically perform with the other leg elevated.

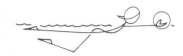

Grip and Jump. With a 25 inch ball pressed firmly between your knees, and using your arms to help pull you along, try jumping movements from the **Dolphin** (p. 82) such as: (1) jump up and down in place, (2) jump forward and backward across the pool, (3) from side to side, (4) jump up and land with your knees alternately to the right, then the left, and/or (5) try several sequences alternating 10 repetitions each of (1) and (4).

FIGURE 9-65

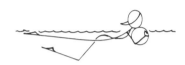

SQUID

Kicking exercises for endurance and for muscles of legs and lower trunk

FIGURE 9-66

GET SET: Stand at one side of the pool in **water at least chest deep.** Hold a 25 to 29 inch beach ball as suggested below.

GO: Kick across several widths of the pool using any of these movements. Or, to keep the action interesting, change to a different style each width. For further variety, you also can do many **Surfbird** movements (p. 144) with a beach ball instead of a kickboard.

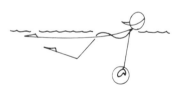

Travel Forward. Move forward in a horizontal position using flutter or breast stroke kicks while holding the ball:

FIGURE 9-67

1. Forward on the surface, elbows straight (Fig. 9-65). For extra arm-firming benefits, push hands down against the ball as you kick.
2. Under your chin (Fig. 9-66). Try pressing down on the ball with your chin to firm your neck.
3. Straight down (Fig. 9-67).
4. Forward on the surface. Bring legs together after every eight kicks, then tuck knees forward at the same time you press arms down to vertical and touch ball to the top of your feet (Fig. 9-68). Reverse the motion, moving ball forward as you extend legs back, then immediately resume kicking. Keep legs together and arms straight as you tuck up and extend.
5. Forward on the surface. Flutter kick 16 times. During the last two kicks, lower legs to vertical, then flutter kick eight times

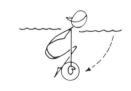

FIGURE 9-68

turning in a circle while swinging the ball along in front (Fig. 9-69). Immediately resume horizontal position and repeat the sequence several times. Kick nonstop as you alternate between horizontal and vertical positions and periodically turn in the opposite direction.

Travel Backward. Move backward by flutter kicking and holding the ball:

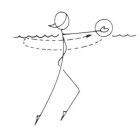

1. Behind your head as if the ball were a pillow, elbows pressed back in the water (Fig. 9-70). Limit the ball size to 25 inches or less because a larger ball can strain the neck by pushing the head too far forward.

FIGURE 9-69

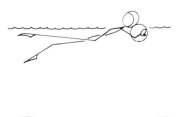

FIGURE 9-70

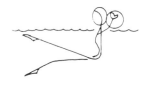

FIGURE 9-71

2. As in version #1. Alternate that kick with kicking in pike position (Fig. 9-71). Progress across the pool using 16 kicks in each position. During pike, keep head and back erect, elbows pressed back. Try to kick toes up to the surface.
3. In front on the surface (Fig. 9-72). As you kick, swing the ball through the surface from side to side. Keep elbows straight and try to swing the ball around to shoulder level at each side (Fig. 9-73).
4. Forward on the surface with legs piked forward. Try to kick up to the ball (Fig. 9-74).

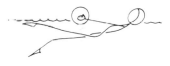

FIGURE 9-72

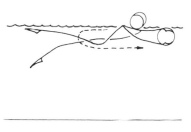

FIGURE 9-73

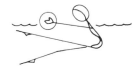

FIGURE 9-74

5. Pressed against the back of your waist, elbows pointing side-ward (Fig. 9-75). Pike legs forward and try to kick up to the surface.
6. Pressed against your buttocks (Fig. 9-76). In other words, sit on the ball with arms down, hands holding sides of ball.
7. Forward on the surface. Move alternately back and forth by kicking backward with your legs piked (Fig. 9-74) and kicking forward on your front with legs extended to the back. Change body position and direction every 16 kicks. Or, to progress slowly across the pool, alternate 8 kicks backward, body piked, with 24 forward kicks, body extended. Arms remain forward the entire time.

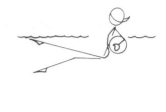

FIGURE 9-75

Travel and Roll. Clasp your arms around one ball by holding it against your chest or hold two balls, one under each arm. Now, flutter or breast stroke kick forward, first on your front, then roll over and continue kicking in the same direction on your back. Repeat this sequence across the pool using 16 kicks in each position. To roll smoothly, flutter kick continuously; for breast stroke kick, roll just as legs come together for the glide. Periodically roll in the opposite direction.

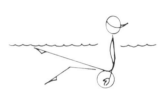

FIGURE 9-76

More Beach Ball Ideas
(for Workouts, Games, Races)

Here are some fun-filled ideas, ranging from easy to hard, that can be done with two or more people. However, many of them can be done by individuals who want to include combinations of beach ball movements in their workouts. (Numbers 5 through 14 are particularly appropriate.) See how they stimulate your imagination for other beach ball movements and combinations.

1. Stand in **waist-deep water** with a partner, each of you holding a 25 inch ball. Then, bend over and press it down to the bottom of the pool. See who can keep it there the longest. *A tip:* To get the ball down, stay over it by holding your head down in the water and kicking hard. An even greater challenge is to do a handstand while holding the ball on the bottom, legs and body straight (Fig. 9-77).
2. With a group of people, stand in **waist-to-chest-deep water** in a circle with every third or fourth person holding a 25 to 29 inch ball. Next, toss the balls to the right from person to person. However, before tossing the ball, each participant

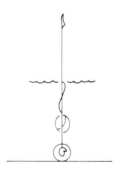

FIGURE 9-77

must first press it beneath the surface. Someone should be appointed the ''caller'' who, at his or her whim, will call out ''change'' to have the balls tossed in the opposite direction.

3. Stand in **waist-to-chest-deep water** facing your partner and hold a ball between you, with arms forward and elbows straight (Fig. 9-78). Now, see who can push the other backward as you both lie front down, heads up, and kick hard using either the flutter or breast stroke kick. Kick 30 times; stand up and catch three breaths, then repeat.

4. If your pool has lane lines on the bottom, you can play this racing game. Start by standing in a line, each person holding a ball forward on the surface. Now, all run forward (Fig. 9-79) and, as you pass each line, push the ball far beneath the surface, then release it, letting it pop out of the water (Fig. 9-80). Quickly catch It and continue across the pool, repeating the push-catch action at each black line. Then, race back to the starting point using one of the methods suggested in #5 or #6 below.

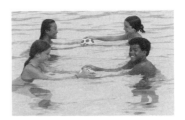

FIGURE 9-78

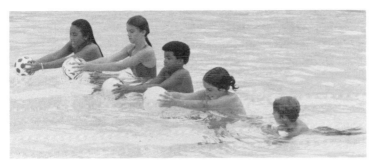

FIGURE 9-79

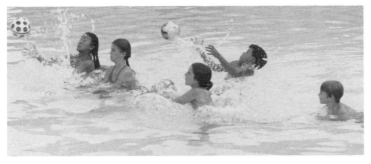

FIGURE 9-80

5. Move back and forth across the pool using your legs as in **Squid** or **Ballyhoo.** Move across using one style and return using another.

6. Move back and forth across the pool poised atop the ball and using your arms as in **Capybara, Diatom,** or **Pink Fairy.** Do each width of the pool in a different style.

7. Combine #6 and #6 above by moving across the pool using your legs; then, return using your arms. This lets you move for longer periods with less fatigue by changing the workload from one muscle group to another.

8. To add even more fun and variety, when using **Squid** or **Ballyhoo** movements, stop midway across the pool and use movements that require stretching, bending, or pushing the ball under the water as in **Sea Moth, Sunfish, Balloon Fish,** or **Shoveler.** Repeat the chosen movement 8 to 15 times. Or, you can jump and twist or hop and stretch as in #9 and #10 below.

9. *Throughout the entire exercise,* hold the ball either (1) overhead with arms straight, (2) on top of your head or against the back of your neck (press elbows back), or (3) straight out in front at shoulder level. Now, jump up and down, landing alternately facing right (Fig. 9-81) then left. To help with the reversing action, twist at the waist and swing your shoulders forcefully around to the side as you land. This Aquacise adds waist exercise and should be done eight times at first. Gradually increase to 15 repetitions to each side.

10. For more waist exercise, try both of these versions: (1) Start with ball overhead, one leg forward, toes at the surface. Now, hop once as you lower the ball toward your toes (Fig. 9-82); hop again as you swing the ball overhead and back (Fig. 9-83). (2) Start with one leg elevated to the side, ball overhead. Hop once as you swing the ball down, turning shoulders toward extended foot (Fig. 9-84). Turn shoulders to face front as you hop again and swing the ball overhead and to the other side (Fig. 9-85). Periodically perform with the other leg elevated and, if you like, omit the hop. Keep knee of elevated leg straight. Use the same repetitions as #9.

11. Walk quickly forward or sideways across the pool while pressing the ball down behind your hips. Press down firmly with the heels of your hands, elbows straight.

12. Walk quickly forward or backward across the pool, holding the ball on the surface in front, elbows straight. Step on one foot, then kick the other leg high to bring toes up to the ball (Fig. 9-86). Repeat the step-kick action, alternating legs.

13. Run forward through the water pushing the ball forward, half submerged, elbows straight (Fig. 9-87). For variety, perform several sequences alternating one width of the pool of #12 with one of #13.

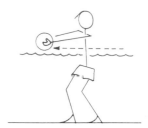

FIGURE 9-81

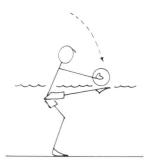

FIGURE 9-82

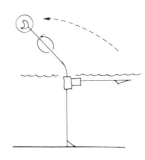

FIGURE 9-83

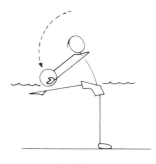

FIGURE 9-84

14. Hold the ball forward on the surface. Lean forward and lift your right leg high to the back, knee straight. Now, take eight hops backward on the left foot; then walk, jog, or flutter kick forward to the starting place. Each time you repeat the sequence, hop backward on the opposite foot.

15. With a partner, face each other and walk sideways across two widths of the pool, tossing the ball back and forth as you go. Then, try it again—this time with one partner moving forward, the other backward.

16. Lie front down and kick forward across the pool holding the ball under your chin as in Fig. 9-66. Then, repeat several times any Aquacise from **Shoveler, Sea Moth,** or **Anchovy.** Finally, jump quickly back to the starting place with the ball held overhead.

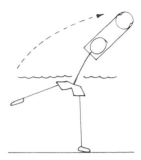

FIGURE 9-85

17. Hold the ball on top of your head, then walk quickly sideways across the pool taking giant steps. Next, toss the ball high into the air and catch it four times. Return to the start by running backward or kicking on your back while holding the ball in one hand. The first person to reach the starting point, stand, and hold the ball on top of her head is the winner.

18. Divide into two teams of three or four participants each and have a medley relay. The first person can kick across and back on her front with the ball held under her chin or straight down (see Figs. 9-66 and 9-67). The second person can run, jump, or leap across two widths holding the ball overhead. The third person can swim two widths on her back with the ball held overhead on the surface. Have the fourth person do **Travel and Roll** (p. 194).

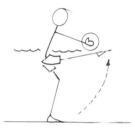

FIGURE 9-86

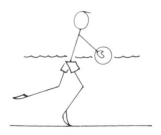

FIGURE 9-87

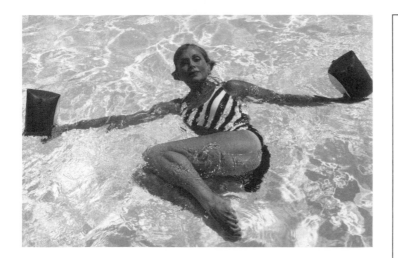

Water wings are simply inflatable swim teaching aids which add more fun and challenge to Water Workouts. They can be used in two ways, (1) hand held for support as described in the "Stretchaway" and "By the Sea" chapters, or (2) with proper caution, worn on the lower legs to intensify many other Aquacises presented later on.

My students and I have tried several types of water wings but none compared in durability, price, and effectiveness to BEMA Schwimflugels (dubbed "floogels"); therefore, throughout this book, BEMA Schwimflugels are synonymous with the term "water wings." Their triangular shape allows them to be slipped on and off easily and there is a larger size available for ages 13 and up. Get them at your local swimming pool supply store or write BEMA, U.S.A., 2015 Weaver Park Drive, Clearwater, FL 33515 for price and availability.

But first, a word of caution to people who want to use "floogels" on their lower legs to intensify the water's resistance and the stretch of Lower Limb Aquacises. Remember!...you can easily capsize with these devices on your legs. Accordingly, don't try them unless you are comfortable in the water and can readily recover from back and front floating positions to an upright standing position. Even then, you may need to practice doing the same with floogels on your legs.

A second word of caution for those with low back problems. In order to get floogels on and off your legs, you must be able to bend forward and lift your knees. Consequently, unless you have a healthy back, avoid these activities at least until you have used some of the other Aquacises to develop and strengthen your lower back muscles. Later, you'll discover that "floogeling" actually strengthens lower back and abdominal muscles. However, in the event you do capsize, protect your lower back by **not** twisting to right yourself. Instead, just relax and float while paddling to the pool ledge. Grasp the ledge, then roll over to your front, tuck up your knees, and straighten your legs down to gain an upright position.

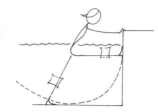

Because floogels on the legs affect balance, also remember to do the Aquacises with your body in alignment. Stand and move tall and pull in your abdomen. Floogels can be kept in place on the legs by inflating them sufficiently and removing any body lotion beforehand. Now, after a good warm-up, you should be ready to start "floogeling."

1. For the easiest start, try "Feather Duster," p. 116-121, a floogel in each hand and/or wear one on each wrist. These are excellent Aquacises particularly for people with arthritis. Next, observe the cautions previously described, and try some of the following:

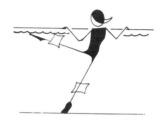

2. "Shape-Up Aquacises" for the lower limbs. For increased flexibility, allow the floogel to gently lift your limb. To tone and strengthen, swing your legs with more force and through a larger range of motion.

3. With floogels on the lower legs, try some "Shape-Up Aquacises" for the trunk, such as **Turnstone, Naiad, Triggerfish, Jollytail, Pipefish. Exclude** those that hyper-extend the low back by moving both legs simultaneously, such as **Sea Squirt, Ribbonfish,** and **Knifefish,** unless abdominal and lower back muscles are conditioned for these strenuous Aquacises.

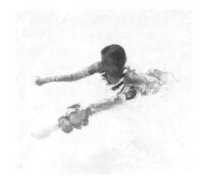

4. "Walk, Jog, Jump, Hop, and Kick Aquacises," especially jumping and hopping movements where floogels give added lift. Pay extra attention to body alignment to stay upright and get the most out of each motion. Also, keep hands in the water for balance and for pulling yourself along. Two favorites in these groups are **Leap** and **Run Upstream.**

5. For increased flexibility, try some slow leg movements from the "Stretchaway" chapter, especially **Mudskipper, Fallfish** variation **Fall Side, Feet Apart; Petticoat Fish, Pumpkinseed; Lady of the Waters; Tip-Up;** and **Sea Whip.** Exclude **Nudibranch** in the beginning.

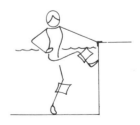

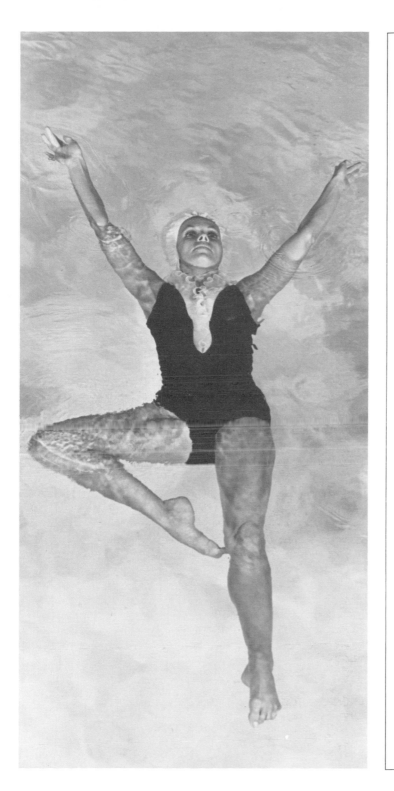

Part IV

PLANNING YOUR WATER WORKOUTS™

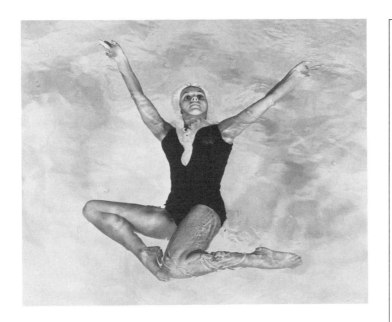

Program A

Build your fitness sessions around the forceful, sweeping movements of "Shape-Up Aquacises" and the brisk, lively "Walk, Jog, Jump, Hop, and Kick Aquacises." Then, finish each session with "Stretchaway" movements.

1. Warm up gradually by walking through the shallow water, or lightly jog, kick, swim, or breathe and bob until you feel pleasantly invigorated.
2. Choose three or more Shape-ups from each of the following groups: Upper Limbs (p. 20), Trunk (p. 36), and Lower Limbs (p. 56). Do them in any order you prefer and, unless advised otherwise, work up until you can perform each a minimum of 15 to a maximum of 25 times. For a balanced program, select a variety of Shape-Ups that collectively move the limbs forward, backward, and sideward. If you like, either supplement or replace Upper Limb and/or Trunk Shape-Ups with "Paddle Aquacises" (p. 126).
3. Intersperse Shape-Ups with "Walk, Jog, Jump, Hop, and Kick Aquacises" (p. 72). "Kickboarding" (p. 138), or some swimming strokes. In addition, use these brisk movements nonstop (in any combination) for longer durations to improve your cardiovascular fitness. See "Why and How to Aquacise Aerobically" for details.

203

4. Take an extra five minutes or so at the end of your session to unwind with "Stretchaway" movements (p. 98). Or, just float or "marinate" while the water's reverse gravitational effect helps your circulation return to normal. In the near gravity-free water, the traditional cool down using less vigorous activity is not mandatory because blood does not tend to pool in the lower extremities as it does on land when vigorous activity is stopped abruptly.

Program B

Build your fitness sessions around "Kickboard Kapers" or, if you Aquacise five or six days a week, substitute a kickboard session for two of those days.

1. Warm up gradually by walking through the shallow water, or lightly jog, kick, swim, or breathe and bob until you feel pleasantly invigorated.
2. Choose four or more movements from the **Crocodile** group (p. 150). Do them in any order you prefer using the suggested number of repetitions. In addition, do movements for the lower limbs from the **Balloon Fish** (p. 178) by substituting a kickboard for the ball. Or, do several Lower Limb Shape-Ups.
3. After learning to balance on the board in the required positions (during your warm-up is ideal), choose several of the more energetic movements from these groups; **Clown-fish** (p. 153), **Flounder** (p. 155), **Angelfish** (p. 158), and/or **Swan** (p. 161).
4. Intersperse #2 and #3 above with any movements from "Kickboarding" (p. 138) and/or "More Kickboard Ideas" (p. 166). Or, use these brisk movements nonstop for longer trips to increase your aerobic fitness. See "Why and How to Aquacise Aerobically" for details.
5. Complete your session by stretching or improving your balance and coordination with less vigorous movements from the **Crocodile** (such as **Pull Down in Back** or **Single Arm Press Down** and their variations), **Flounder, Angelfish, Moon-fish** (p. 160), and/or **Flamingo** (p. 164).

Program C

Build your fitness sessions around the widely diversified "Beach Ball Aquacises" or, if you Aquacise five or six days a week, try using beach ball sessions for two of those days.

1. Warm up gradually by walking through the shallow water, or lightly jog, kick, swim, or breathe and bob until you feel pleasantly invigorated.
2. Choose four or more Beach Ball Aquacises from each of the following groups: **Shoveler** (p. 173), **Balloon Fish** (p. 178), and **Stinker** (p. 182), or **Capybara** (p. 185). If you like, also include some repetitions of **Mussel** (p. 173) and **Anchovy** (p. 176). Do them in any order you prefer using the suggested number of repetitions.
3. Intersperse the above categories with "More Beach Ball Ideas" (choose among #3 through #18, p. 195) and/or individual movements from **Squid** (p. 192) or **Ballyhoo** (p. 190). Or, you can use any combination of these movements nonstop for longer voyages to further increase your cardio-vascular fitness. "Why and How to Aquacise Aerobically" tells how.
4. Allow extra time at the end of your session to gain additional body tone, flexibility, balance, and coordination with se-lected movements from **Sea Moth** (p. 177), **Sunfish** (p. 180), **Diatom** (p. 187), and/or **Pink Fairy** (p. 188).

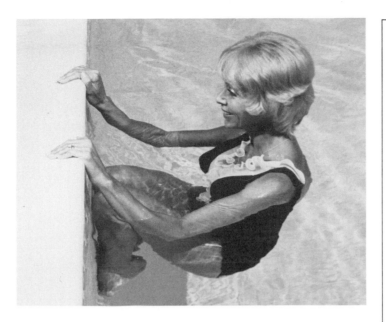

You have two feedback mechanisms to help you adjust your exercise intensity to make it just right for you. One is a subjective response, the other physiological. The first response is your perception of exertion, a "subjective feeling of effort and fatigue," during which you naturally "regulate the work intensity in relation to how hard the work feels."[11] This sensation is related to workload and heart rate. The physiological response is your heartbeat which you can monitor yourself. Pulse monitoring, as described in this chapter, enables you to maintain a level of exertion that will ensure cardiovascular benefits without overexertion. It is also a valuable tool for learning how to "use" the water to get the most out of Aquacising and for confirming the accuracy of your perceived exertion.[12]

During exercise, your heartbeat reflects your moment-to-moment physiological state by telling you exactly how hard you are working. Fatigue, overly warm water (ideal is between 78° and 82°), or a low fitness level all increase the effort of your exercise so that you actually work less to bring your pulse to target level. On the other hand, as your fitness improves, you will have to work harder to reach that same target level.

Most physicians and physical educators consider aerobic (cardiovascular) fitness the most critical component of total

[11] G. Borg, "Perceived Exertion as an Indicator of Somatic Stress," *Scand. J. Rehab. Med.,* 2(1970), 92–98.

[12] Recognition of the degree of increased heartbeat and breathlessness which indicates your aerobic target zone and thereby eliminates the need for frequent pulse counting.

fitness. Essentially, regular aerobic activity will (1) lower your blood pressure if you are hypertensive, (2) lower your triglyceride and cholesterol levels, (3) lower your heart rate both at rest and during exercise, (4) enable you to exercise longer and harder with less effort and recover from exortion more quickly, (5) help convert body fat to firm, lean tissue, and (6) delay the aging process.

The extent of these benefits will depend on the intensity, frequency, and the duration of your fitness sessions. To get the most out of them, (1) perform your Workouts with sufficient intensity to keep your pulse in your target zone, (2) Aquacise a minimum of three nonconsecutive days each week, (3) move continuously, after a several-minute warm-up, for a minimum of 20 minutes, and (4) progressively increase your workload by using the suggestions on page 12.

Three heart rates are important in your quest for improved cardiovascular fitness. But, before we address them, let's learn how to take a pulse by placing the first three fingers of one hand lightly (1) just forward of the vertical muscle at the side of your neck or (2) at the base of your thumb joint just inside your wrist bone. Generally, students prefer to use the first method when exercising in the water. If you have difficulty finding your pulse, try amplifying it by walking briskly. Once you know how to locate your pulse, time it as noted below.

RESTING HEART RATE (RHR). Your RHR tells you how hard your heart is working at rest. Average RHRs for women are 75–80, for men 72–76. To determine your RHR, take your pulse for one minute on three consecutive days, then compute the average. Take it sometime before noon after sitting quietly for at least 15 minutes. Even if your RHR is in the low to normal range, you should still try to reduce it further for all of the reasons stated earlier. However, it usually takes a minimum of four weeks of aerobic training to begin to lower your RHR.

EXERCISE HEART RATE (EHR). To compute your exercise target zone, use the method supported by the American Heart Association. Subtract your age from 220 and multiply the answer by .70 to get the number of beats/minute for your *minimum* EHR and by .85 to get your *maximum* EHR.

Example

220	220
$\underline{-40}$ = age	$\underline{-40}$ = age
180	180
$\underline{\times.70}$	$\underline{\times.85}$
126.00 or 126 beats/min.	153.00 or 153 beats/min.
minimum EHR	*maximum* EHR

As you Aquacise aerobically, adjust the intensity of your movements to keep your level of exertion in this range by moving more vigorously for a short time, then easing up as you begin to tire. Later on, you will be able to sustain the higher level for longer periods. It's worth noting that target zone figures may vary considerably from one person to another, so adjust to higher or lower rates according to your exercise capacity.[13] It's also worth noting that beginning Aquacisers are sometimes unable to get their EHR up to the minimum target level. This temporary situation is eliminated when students learn which movements elevate the heart rate (vigorous movements of large muscle groups) and how to put forth more effort. Often, the EHR can be brought up to target by doing standing, or upright, movements in shallower water (not less than waist deep).

Remember that the EHR is affected by the speed, force, and range of your movements. As you work with the Aquacises in your program, you will increase both your strength and flexibility, enabling you to put forth more effort and achieve higher EHRs. The stronger you are, the more speed and force you can apply, and the greater your flexibility, the farther you can swing your arms and legs against the water's resistance for increased workload and EHR. Furthermore, arm movements such as those in "Upper Limb Shape-Ups" generally produce slightly lower EHRs than the vigorous leg movements found in "Lower Limb" and "Trunk Shape-Ups"; "Walk, Jog, Jump, Hop, Kick Aquacises"; "Kickboarding"; "More Kickboard Kapers"; and from the "Beach Ball" chapter, **Squid, Ballyhoo,** and "More Beach Ball Ideas" (#3 through #18).

If you are Aquacising in a class, your instructor can tell you when to start and stop counting your pulse. When exercising alone, place a stop watch and towel on the pool deck within easy reach. (If your indoor pool has a pace clock on the wall, so much the better.) In the beginning, take your pulse every three to five minutes. For accuracy, timing should be done as soon as possible after exercise ceases because at that time your pulse drops rapidly. Once you find your pulse, time it for ten seconds and multiply the number of beats by six. First, locate your pulse with one hand then, with the other hand, click on your stop watch and begin counting your heartbeats.

---

[13]Overexertion can cause nausea, insomnia, next-day fatigue, breathlessness lasting more than 10 minutes after exercise, or target-rate heart action 5 to 10 minutes after exercise. If so, ease up during subsequent sessions. If you experience chest pain during or following the session, abnormal heart rhythm, dizziness, or gastrointestinal upset, see your physician before resuming your program.

RECOVERY HEART RATE: At the end of your session, stay in the water for an additional five minutes or so to give your circulatory system a chance to return to more normal levels. Before leaving the water, your heart rate should be down to 120 beats/minute or less. When you are ready to take this final measurement, count for 15 seconds at which time your count should be down to 30 or less (30 × 4 = 120 beats/min.). If it's higher, stay in the water a few extra minutes and then time it again.

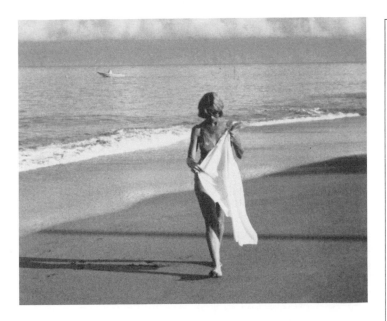

Chapter 13
"BY THE SEA, BY THE SEA, BY THE BEAUTIFUL SEA. . ." (AND LAKE)

If you have ever experienced a swim in the ocean, you know the joyous, buoyant feeling that salt water provides. Similarly, that same buoyancy can be a big plus when you try your Aquacises in the ocean. Many Aquacises can be used "as is," while others can be used with simple adaptations in either ocean or lake. However, the most important elements are calm, inviting water and a smooth bottom. In addition, you should be able to (1) face and back float and recover to a standing position, (2) tread water, and (3) swim well enough to easily reach shore should swimming be necessary.

To make your nonpool Aquacises even more enjoyable, I recommend three types of easy-to-pack equipment: a pair of snug-fitting rubber beach shoes to protect your feet from rough underwater surfaces; a set of Aquacise paddles to enhance arm movements and swimming strokes; and a pair of adult-size swim wings in the place of your kickboard to use during swim kicks and to aid balance during Lower Limb and Trunk Shape-Ups. Also, if you are in an area with clear waters and abundant sea life, go prepared to snorkel and see first hand some of the beautiful creatures the Aquacises were named after. All you need are a well-fitted face mask and snorkel tube which you should buy and test at home beforehand. Swim fins will add to your mobility but these can usually be rented at a modest fee at your resort hotel or a dive shop. Even if you have never snorkeled before, don't be deterred. A few minutes with a local instructor will pay big dividends and enable you to discover the kaleidoscopic world that exists just beneath the surface, especially around coral reefs.

Following is a rundown of the various categories of Aquacises and how they may be used in open-water areas.

UPPER LIMB SHAPE-UPS: Use any movements except those that require the solid support of a pool ledge, although most **Oarfish** variations can be done while floating free. **Jacknife Fish** and **Anemone** are especially fun and beneficial because of their added hip and thigh benefits. If you like, hold a swim wing (or paddle) in each hand or wear a wing on each wrist.

TRUNK SHAPE-UPS: Nearly all of the standing movements may be used, especially if you stabilize yourself by holding an inflated swim wing in each hand for support, arms sideward, hands in the water. Omit side-slant or suspended movements requiring the solid support of a pool ledge. The exceptions are: **Croaker**—hold both swim wings in one hand and lean in that direction with the body straight as if supported by a pool ledge. When tucking up knees, try to touch your feet to that hand. **Jollytail**—hold arms sideward and stand in tiptoe-deep water. Jump up lightly each time you lift your knees. **Ribbon-fish**—hold arms sideward and tuck knees to alternate elbows, rolling onto your side to do so. Keep legs close to the surface. **Anglerfish**—hold arms sideward and swing them through the water as necessary for stability. **Dragonfly, Scud, Sand Bug,** and **Barnacle**—hold arms sideward. **Naiad** and **Triggerfish**—hold both wings in one hand and exercise the opposite limb(s). **Triggerfish** (**Touch Across** variation)—touch toes to opposite hand.

LOWER LIMB SHAPE-UPS: Nearly all of these movements can be used except those done from side-slant or suspended positions (also omit **Push—Pull** variations from **Daphnia** and **Grunt**). For the others, balance yourself by standing erect, arms sideward, and preferably with a swim wing in each hand for stability. Here are some helpful tips: **Jewelfish**—do the basic movement with arms in a wide V, hands at the surface, then kick up to fingers. **Swordfish, Snapper** (**Snap Side** variation), **Hip-popotamus** (basic movement and variations)—hold arms sideward and kick up to fingers. **Water Witch**—hold both wings in one hand and exercise the opposite limbs. **Snapper** (basic movement)—during the backward motion, lift heel toward buttocks.

WALK, JOG, JUMP, HOP, KICK: Moving parallel to the shore, try as many of these movements as you can remember. Movements from the **Salmon** group are fun to do in deeper water while suspended vertically, arms sideward, with a swim wing in each hand.

STRETCHAWAY: Omit most movements in this group because they require the support of a pool ledge. However, all movements in **Feather Duster** are ideal for use in open waters. Furthermore, many in that group can be done in salt water without any floating supports.

PADDLE AQUACISES: All movements may be used except **Fancy Sea Robin.** Do the basic **Sea Robin** and **Platypus** standing erect, although **Platypus** should still be done with one leg forward.

KICKBOARD KAPERS: Use any of your basic swim kicks and variations (**Water Boatman** and **Surfbird**) with your arms forward at the surface, a swim wing in each hand. In salt water, many people can dispense with floating supports and kick with arms forward at the surface or with hands on the hips. For obvious reasons, forego "Aquabatics" unless you have a kickboard.

BEACH BALL: If you have a beach ball, you can use all movements in open waters except the **Stinker** and, unless the water is very calm, the **Pink Fairy.**

GLOSSARY OF WATER CREATURES

ANEMONE is one of the 6,100 species of marine (saltwater) animals having a flower-like form (Anthoza class). It is found worldwide in a variety of colors and forms, mostly in the subaqua gardens of warm, shallow waters. Sea anemones have stubby, cylindrical bodies capable of changing shape in a variety of ways as the situation requires. At the upper end is a central, all-purpose opening encircled by one or more rows of graceful, yet poisonous tentacles. At the other end is a smooth, muscular disc for attaching itself to rocks or thrusting into sand or crevices. While most sea anemones stay fixed in one spot, some can slide slowly on their base. Others can creep along by lying on their trunk and alternately contracting and extending it. When threatened, some species (e.g., *Stomphia*) can even detach from their mooring and swim away using a series of jerky, bending movements. Other species hitch a ride on the shells of hermit crabs where they trade the protection of their stinging tentacles for leftover tidbits from the crab's meal. Sometimes the crab lifts the anemone onto its shell. At other times the anemone gets there alone by cartwheeling end over end in slow motion onto the shell. Once the foot is attached, it straightens up, ready for a ride.

ANGELFISH (family Chaetodontidae) are seen in pairs or small groups in the sunlit waters of coral reefs. They shimmer with extravagant colors and patterns that vary among species and also among their young. Although inquisitive, they are unruffled by the presence of snorkelers or scuba divers and often swim just out of reach — tilting to one side to get a better look. Some young angels set up cleaning stations on a rock or coral head, then do a wiggly "dance" to advertise their grooming services to other fish.

ANGLERFISH are a group of at least 200 species of grotesque, yet fascinating fish found at every depth in tropical and temperate seas. Generally, they are shaped like squat blobs bedecked with warty protuberances and flaps of skin for camouflage. All have various fishing pole and lure arrangements for attracting unwary prey. The fishing pole is often an extension of the first dorsal fin which is on the snout. The lure, which may be luminescent, looks like a tender morsel of food that is slowly waved back and forth. Sometimes the anglerfish just lies in wait for a prospective meal, its cavernous mouth agape. At other times, the angler waits until an inquisitive fish hesitates to investigate then it snaps open its mouth and the inrushing water pulls the hapless victim with it. This action is quicker than a human eye can see. Another bizarre episode in the life of the anglerfish occurs among some deep sea species who carry the idea of togetherness to the extreme. The male, often only 1/2 inch long, sinks his teeth into the much larger female. Eventually his mouth fuses to her skin and all his organs degenerate until he is transformed into a mere sperm-producing machine, nourished by what has become a shared blood system.

ARCHERFISH include five species of the family Toxotidae that inhabit brakish and freshwater areas between southern Asia and northern Australia. They are nature's finned sharpshooters, famous for their ability to shoot jets of water as far as nine feet above the surface to bring down insects from low-hanging vegetation. (Baby archerfish begin to "shoot" when about one inch long.)

BALLOON FISH (family Diondontidae) is also fittingly named globefish and porcupinefish. It inhabits tropical or subtropical waters of mangrove swamps, coral reefs, and sandy bays worldwide and its young are often found among pastures of floating vegetation. It has large eyes and a typical 1 to 2½-foot long, fish-shaped body covered with sharp spines that lie flat. However, when alarmed, it inflates like a balloon by drawing in water (or air when out of the water) and raises its spines. This defensive tactic makes the fish unappetizing to predators but makes its fins nearly useless until its plump shape returns to normal.

BALLYHOO, or *Hemiramphus brasiliensis*, belongs to the family Exocoetidae and is related to garfish and needlefish. It is an inshore species, ranging from New England to Brazil and throughout the Gulf of Mexico and Caribbean. It has a slim, 18 inch long body with long, slender uneven jaws, the lower being the longest. The tip of its lower jaw and the upper tail lobe are both orange and its underside is silvery with dark green or blue black. Swift and playful, the ballyhoo swims in schools close to the surface, sometimes skipping and skittering across it.

BARNACLE. The acorn barnacle is the most widely known of this group of highly modified crustaceans known as the cirripides. Clusters of them live, each in a limey shell, anchored head down to the substrate. They feed on tiny animals and organic fragments swept toward their mouths with bristle-fringed appendages. Barnacle eggs develop within the parent's body and hatch into microscopic larvae. After progressing through several stages, the tiny shrimp-like beings, now encased in light bivalve shells, are ready to settle down and cement themselves permanently to substructures such as rocks, wood, and even turtles and crabs. One, the goose barnacle, *Lepas fascicularis,* prefers to roam by hanging from its stalk in bunches from a raft—head up, legs dangling, and ready to scoop up tiny morsels. Any conveyance will do, from the underside of ships to floating bottles and light bulbs.

BOOBY (family Sulidae) is an extraordinary "aqua-bird," a creature of both tropical air and sea. Like the pelican, the booby has an inflatable air sac under its skin to provide buoyancy and to cushion the impact of striking the water in the pursuit of prey. When searching for food, it sometimes flies high into the air and plummets headfirst into the water; then without pausing it arcs back to the surface. However, when it surfaces, the fish it has caught is very often hijacked by a crafty frigate bird. Also, its large webbed feet make it as ungainly on land as a human walking in swim fins, but booby still paddles efficiently at the surface.

BUTTERFLYFISH. Marine butterflyfish live in the fairy-land of coral reefs and belong to the same family (Chaetodontidae) as marine angelfish. Their 6 to 8-inch long, oval- to pancake-shaped bodies are marked with a variety of striking colors and patterns. There are a wide variety of butterflyfish, all of them agile and graceful swimmers. They characteristically swim in pairs and have their own feeding territory which they defend against intrusion.

There are also "sea butterflies" known as pteropods that are actually tiny snails whose feet are flattened like thin paddles or wings which they flap constantly to fly horizontally or spiral upward through the water. Most don't exceed ½ inch in length, and many have delicate transparent shells while others are naked. They occur in vast numbers among the plankton of temperate and tropical seas.

CAPYBARA (*Hydrochoerus hydrochaeris*). This tail-less, partially webfooted animal is the largest member of the rodent family, often growing to a length of four feet. Essentially aquatic and an excellent swimmer, its eyes, ears, and nostrils are mounted on top of its head so that it can hide in the water. Capybaras live in groups by rivers and lakes in tropical South America and are easily tamed by the adventurous.

CLOWNFISH, or anemone fish, belong to the family Pomacentridae along with various other small marine fish found in tropical Atlantic and Indo-Pacific waters and collectively known as damsel-fish. Most are lively, brightly colored, and live around coral reefs. Several species of clownfish, of the genus *Amphirprion,* are all from the Indo-Pacific and are so named because of their vivid "swimsuits." In fact clownfish species are so similarly marked that it is often difficult to tell one from another, though generally they sport bright hues of rust-red with bold vertical white stripes. Their alternate name, anemone fish, derives from their symbiotic relationship with various species of anemones. The clownfish takes refuge among the anemone's poisonous tentacles to sleep, escape danger, or to eat—sometimes even pulling food from the anemone's mouth. To reciprocate, the clownfish feeds bits of food to its landlord and, some believe, even lures other fish into its host's deadly arms.

CORMORANTS belong to a family of birds (Phalacrocoracidae) comprising 30 species of which the Great or Common Cormant, *Phalacrocorax carbo,* is the largest and most widely distributed. It has a long body, neck, and beak, and short legs with webbed feet. It also is a fast swimmer, zooming along low in the water, head out. The Great Cormorant is a very efficient underwater hunter, first executing a graceful, splashless surface dive, then gliding along under the surface propelled by its powerful legs. Because it is intelligent and easily tamed, this cormorant has been trained to fish, both as a regular sport during the reign of Charles I of England, and as a means of livelihood by fishermen, particularly the Japanese. Though now only a tourist attraction, this method of fishing was used for over a thousand years. Each of the fisherman's prized cormorants wore a special collar which was attached to a leash, though the tamest birds were said to require none. The neck ring was sized to allow the bird to swallow the smallest fish and, when his gullet filled with larger ones, he was pulled to the boat where he disgorged his catch, accepted a "thank you" tidbit, and was off again for another round of fishing.

CROAKERS belong to a large family (Sciaenidae) of fish, many of which live in tropical and temperate seas. While many fish make sounds, croakers are particularly vocal, producing humming, purring, croaking, and booming noises, even, some people say, sounds akin to a melody. Most often the sounds are made by rapid vibrations of muscles that run from their abdomen to their branched swim bladder which acts as a sounding board. Often the sounds are quite loud, clearly discernable from above the surface. These fish are also called drums because of their ability to produce a drumming noise. *Nibea*, a species found in Japanese waters, forms schools of a million or more fish which are able to synchronize their drumming.

DAPHNIA, a flea-size spark of life belonging to the order Cladocera, is one of 26,000 species in the diverse class of crustaceans. *Daphnia* are most frequently found in fresh water though some are marine animals. Their heads protrude from delicate transparent shells that reveal tiny internal organs and a miniscule heart. A *Daphnia* propels itself through the water with long, plumed antennae — one flick of the antennae provides needed lift, then the *Daphnia* begins to sink until it flicks again.

DIATOMS are single-celled algae, sometimes referred to as microscopic "veggies" of the sea. Each of the 25,000 species is encased in a finely etched silica shell resembling an intricate opal pill box. Like snowflakes, no two are the same. Diatoms are thought to be the most important plants on earth; by the teeming trillions they bob and glide through the sunlit waters of the world, photosynthesizing sunlight into food for vegetarians ranging from minute krill and copepods to humpback whales, and releasing oxygen into the atmosphere for all of us to breathe.

DIPPER, or water ouzel, is one of five species of birds belonging to the family Cinclidae. It is able to dive into swiftly moving streams and swim underwater or walk on the bottom searching for insect prey, mollusks, tiny fish, and crustaceans. Parents build mossy nests on ledges of mountain streams or waterfalls which provide a constant fine spray for the babies and probably serve as an effective water-introduction course.

DISCUS (*Symphsodon discus*) is one of 600 species of freshwater fish of the family Cichlidae which are known for their beauty and interesting behavior. Discus is named after its circular shape and is found in rivers of the Amazon basin. These fish are especially attentive parents, laying their eggs on submerged leaves or a rock which they have carefully cleaned with their mouths. Both parents take turns aerating the eggs with their fins and then take each hatchling in their mouths to another surface to attach it by a short thread. After another 60 hours of "fin fanning," the youngsters begin swimming close to the parents while they "nurse" for a few days on a special protein substance found on the parents' sides.

DRAGONFLIES have two pair of glassy, irridescent wings that swiftly sweep them low over the water then rocket them skyward and back again. Though harmless to humans, they are predatory insects which are beneficial because of their insatiable appetite for midges and mosquitoes. After mating in flight, the female either embeds her eggs in aquatic plants or repeatedly skims the surface of the water with her abdomen to deposit her eggs which settle to the bottom or adhere to submerged vegetation. The resulting nymphs, with gills for breathing under water, are awkward, ugly, and voracious carnivores. But, after moulting a dozen or so times, they are ready to leave their watery nursery, and climb to the surface. Following one last moult, they take their first breath of air and soar skyward, thus linking water to air.

FALLFISH, or *Semotilus corporalis*, is one of many species of freshwater minnows and the largest in eastern North America, ranging from southern Canada southward to Virginia and westward to the Applachians. It is said to be named for its tendency to dwell at the base of waterfalls. The smaller male, which at times reaches a length of 1½ feet, prepares for spawning by digging a depression into which the female deposits her eggs. Afterward, the male covers them with a large mound (often six feet across and three feet high) constructed of carefully selected stones up to three inches in diameter which he pushes into place or carries in his mouth.

FANFISH (family Bramidae). Of the Bramidae family, one species (*Pteraclis velifera*) is a two foot long fish found in oceans in the southern hemisphere. It is silver with dark blue fins and pale turquoise spots at the back of its body. It also has unusual dark blue eyes with silvery irises and a turned down mouth that gives it a disgruntled look. However, its most remarkable features are two huge fanshaped fins—the upper one extending from the head to the forked tail fin and the lower one from just under the chin to the tail fin.

FEATHER DUSTER (family Sabellidae). Easily mistaken for a tiny flower, the feather duster is actually an elegant worm that constructs a tubular dwelling in limestone rocks or coral from which it extends frilly, brightly colored tentacles. These serve as gills to collect oxygen and minute morsels of food from the water. The largest specimens are best seen underwater from a distance, because this illusive creature's sensitive tentacles withdraw in a flash when they perceive a shadow or vibration. There are several species of tube worms having various plumes and colors.

FIREFLY (*Cypridinia hilgendorfi*) is an ostracod (a type of small crustacean) and one of at least a dozen that sparkle with brilliant luminesence. The firefly which is found in Japanese seas glows with an intense blue light when the water is agitated. A few, shaken up in a test tube of water, emit enough light for a human to read by. It is believed they produce this light to scare away their enemies.

FLATFISH comprise a group of six families containing nearly 500 species of mostly bottom-dwelling marine fish of the order Pleuronectiformes. They are found worldwide and many are familiar food fishes including turbot, sole, flounder, and halibut. When first born, a flatfish has a typically fish-like body. However, it soon undergoes a metamorphosis when it turns to one side and flattens out; the air bladder disintegrates and one eye migrates to the other side of the head as does the mouth in varying degrees. Ultimately, the fish adapts to bottom dwelling, lying flat with its eyes uppermost.

FLOUNDER. There are two flounder families belonging to the large community of flatfish. Those of the Bothidae family have eyes on the left side of the head, while the reverse is true of the Pleuronectidae family. Flounders have adapted to both

salt and fresh water and all but the halibut live on the sea floor. They are considered masters of disguise, able to quickly change the color of their nearly round bodies to match the bottom, whether it is made up of sand, pebbles, or even dark mud.

GOBY. Gobies are among fishdom's peewees, most ranging from one to two inches long. The adult *Pandaka pygmaea* of the Philippines is the smallest of all fish, only one-half inch long. Most of the nearly 500 species of gobies (family Gobiidae) are brightly colored shallow water fishes that live in temperate and tropical seas. They are poor swimmers, so they use their tails and pectoral fins to spurt among the rocks and coral. Also, many have joined pelvic fins that form a sucker to anchor themselves to the substrate. While their life styles are diverse, most gobies stay close to a safe retreat, often sharing it with strange roommates. For instance, the goby *Clevelandia ios* holes up with various crustaceans. It reputedly places its larger pieces of food near a crab, waits while the crab tears it apart, then snacks on the smaller morsels. Another live-in odd couple is the blind goby *Typhlogobius californiensis* and the crab *Callianassa affinis*. The goby is completely dependent on the crab to create currents of water that draw tiny organisms to their grotto. In the Caribbean there is the well-known neon cleaner goby *Gobiosoim oceanons*. After a pair "sets up shop" on a coral ledge, larger fish queue up to have their parasites removed. This not only provides the gobies with free treats, but also immunity from their otherwise predatory clients.

GRIBBLE (*Limnoria lignorum*) is a minikin crustacean (about 1/8 inch long) that believes in "strength in numbers." Huge groups of greedy gribbles are found happily boring their way through floating or submerged pilings and driftwood. While some people consider them pests, others might consider their act a noble gesture since they destroy material that could otherwise endanger navigation.

GRUNIONS are long, slender marine fish (family Atherinidae), sometimes called silversides because of the silver band running along their sides. While most grunions live in tropical and temperate seas, the most familiar member of this family lives off the California coast where it is famous for a February to September ritual. Following a new or full moon, thousands of grunions ride the high tides onto the beaches to spawn. Once on the beach, the female anchors herself by her pectoral fins and wriggles vertically into the sand tail first until she is half buried. She then lays 1,000 to 3,000 eggs while the nearest male deposits milt around her.

GRUNTS belong to a large family (Pomadasyidae) of marine fish that live in large schools in the shallow waters and coral reefs of tropical seas. As their name suggests, they produce numerous, very audible sounds both in and out of the water. The sounds, made by grinding their pharyngeal teeth, are amplified by the swim bladder. Mysteriously, some species also display a curious habit of "kissing," an act believed to be associated with courtship rituals. Because of this, some South African and Australian grunts are appropriately named "sweetlips."

HATCHETFISH belong to the family Sternoptychidae and include several species of tiny (1 to 3 inch long) marine fish having iridescent, silvery, hatchet-shaped bodies and narrow tails. They also have clusters of light organs on their undersides which generally glow blue. Hatchetfish live mainly in deep waters of all temperate and tropical seas. Their extremely light weight makes swimming and daily vertical migrations easy. To follow their food supply of plankton, they rise nearly to the surface each night then descend during the day. There are also South American freshwater hatchetfish (family Gasteropelecidae) that live near the surface and can fly short distances by rapidly beating their pectoral fins. However, some authorities believe they leap clear of the water and glide instead. These fish also are said to do a butterfly-like dance during courtship.

HUMBUG (*Dascyllus aruanus*) is a type of damselfish of the family Pomacentridae. It is also called Banded Humbug because its beautiful pearly white body is striped with vertical bands. Humbugs are agile and graceful swimmers and are often found by the hundreds gliding among branching coral reefs. They are very territorial—each male guards his "personal" coral branch, but also recognizes his neighbors' boundaries. Males guard the eggs until hatched.

HUMUHUMU is short for Humuhumunukunukuapuaa, the famous Hawaiian name given to two similar triggerfish of the genus *Rhinecanthus*. In Hawaiian, it means "to fit pieces together." While the

coloration and markings differ, both species are striking and have oblong, compressed bodies typical of the triggerfish family (Balistidae). One species, *aculeatus*, has such bright, abstract markings that it has been dubbed the Picasso fish. Some humuhumu, which live among fairyland coral reefs of the Indo-Pacific, are said to grunt like pigs when taken from the water.

HYDRAS are freshwater animals that masquerade as tiny plants either by dwelling on stems or hanging head down on the surface film of the water. They have soft, tubular bodies with a single opening at one end surrounded by several tentacles. Feeding is done by extending the tentacles and allowing them to wave gently in the water. When a suitable meal brushes against them— perhaps a tiny crustacean or worm—poisonous threads dart from the tentacles, paralyze the prey, then pass it along to the center opening for digestion. Hydras move about slowly by sliding along on a disc-like "foot" or turning end over end in a slow-motion cartwheel. Their namesake is the mythological water serpent, slain by Hercules, that could grow two new heads for every one cut off. Hydras too have an astonishing ability to regenerate, an ability rarely found among animals. If a hydra is cut in half horizontally, the upper part develops a new foot, the lower part new tentacles. Further, a hydra polyp can be cut into 200 pieces, whereupon each piece grows into a new polyp.

JACKNIFE FISH are relatives of drums and croakers (family Sciaenidae) but the best known is *Equetus lanceolatus*, a striking, nocturnal 8 inch long reef fish that lives as an adult in moderately deep waters of Florida and the Caribbean while its young dwell in shallow water. It is usually yellowish with dark, white-rimmed bands and two dorsal fins, the first greatly elongated and erect, and the second extending fringe-like down the back.

JEWELFISH, or *Hemichromis bimaculatus*, belongs to the large Cichlidae family of tropical freshwater fish, and is just one of the more than 200 species in Africa alone. It is a favorite of aquarists because of its interesting but sometimes quarrelsome behavior and its colorful jewel-like appearance, especially during the breeding period. The prospective parents first clean off a hard surface on which the female lays 500 to 700 tiny, pearl-like eggs in rows forming a circular patch. Then they take turns aerating the eggs by fanning them with their pectoral fins. To protect the babies in times of danger, the mother signals them to her by raising and lowering her unpaired fins. However, babies who stray are apt to be escorted back to their nursery stone in their parents' mouths.

JOLLYTAIL, or *Galaxis maculatus,* comes from a unique family of fish (family Galaxiidae) found only in the southern hemisphere. Although they spawn in freshwater estuaries, the young, after hatching, are swept out to sea to spend the winter before returning to fresh water. Jollytails are small, silvery fish with dark spots and rounded fins.

KNIFEFISH *(Nopterus chitala)* belongs to the family Notopteridae and inhabits freshwater areas of tropical Africa and southeast Asia. By day, it is often found suspended at an angle close to the surface. Its 3 foot long, hump-backed body is earth toned with light rings enclosing dark spots that resemble portholes along each side near its tail. It also has a chiffon-like anal fin extending from behind the throat along its underside and converging with its tail fin in an unbroken line around its tapered rear end. By undulating this fin in gentle waves, the fish moves forward or backward with equal agility. In addition, when swimming at moderate speeds, its posterior also swings from side to side as if "wagging its tail."

LADY OF THE WATERS is one of several common names for the Tricolored Heron, *Egretta tricolor,* a graceful, elegant heron that fishes in the summer in shallow waters off the coasts of Louisiana and Texas. Its name is derived from its dainty, feminine mannerisms both in and near the water. It sometimes strides slowly along looking for its quarry but often, with its wings outstretched, prances about lightly—apparently to stir up the water and bring a prospective minnow or fish meal closer to the surface.

LOON. Common Loons *(Gavia immer)* or Great Northern Divers are large, solitary waterbirds with dark plumage boldly marked with patterns of white dots and stripes. They summer alone or in family groups in the northern states, Canada, and Greenland, treading gracefully across clear, mirror-smooth lakes that echo with their long, melancholy calls. In winter they migrate to salt-water areas along southern coasts. They are fast swimmers and can submerge instantly by diving. When hunting for fish and crabs, they dive underwater (often for a minute, and up to three minutes under stress) using their powerful webbed feet and added wing action when needed. Loons also are deep divers, some having been caught in fishing nets 200 feet down. Though well adapted for swimming, these birds cannot stand on land because their legs are placed too far back on their bodies. However, this apparently is forgotten when (according to *Life Histories of North American Birds*) they play a game by running swiftly, with wings half outstretched, side by side in pairs on the surface of the water. After running about a quarter mile, they wheel around and retrace their path to the starting point. This footrace is repeated over and over with only a short breather between races. Playtime apparently ends with a congratulatory "loony" tune.

MARLIN are popular sporting fish of the family Istiophoridae and are found worldwide in tropical and temperate seas. They are powerful as well as graceful, and are among the fastest predators in the sea, sometimes reaching 50 mph. Their swiftness is aided by elongated, streamlined bodies that have long, spear-like snouts, grooves for folding fins into, and powerful, deeply-forked tails. They are also known for their ability to leap high above the water, especially when hooked.

MOONFISH *(Lampris guttatus)* is also known as opah. It is a large, spectacularly colored marine fish found in the midwaters of all tropical and warm temperate seas. Its long, deep, and round body has a brilliant metallic sheen—dark blue on the back and shading to silver on the sides. Lighter, sequin-like spots dot its body while its fins (and edible flesh) are red.

MUDSKIPPER is a common name for a family of goby-like fish that live mainly in brackish water and mangrove swamps in the Indo-Pacific. It is a small, Disneyesque fish that thinks it's a frog and has large eyes on top of its head to see simultaneously in opposite directions. It is named after its habit of leaving the water and pulling itself along on strong pectoral fins, or rearing up on its tail fin and taking foot-high leaps across sand or mudflats in pursuit of insects and small crustaceans. Mudskippers can store gulps of air in a spongy cavity near each gill, enabling them to breathe during terrestrial forays. However, when not traveling about, they frequently perch on rocks and dangle their tails in the water.

MUSKRAT (*Ondata zibethica*) is essentially a freshwater animal that feeds on aquatic vegetation and zooms through the water using its limbs and powerful beaver-like tail. It is well known in North America and Canada and builds either a grass house cemented with mud or a burrow with two entrances, one above and the other below the surface.

MUSSEL. Mussels are bivalve (twin-shelled) mollusks that make their homes anchored to the substrate in great numbers and come into being in a fascinating way. Reproduction takes place by the uniting of eggs and milt that adults release into the sea in prodigious quantities. Between high and low tides, a fertilized egg is transformed into a minute ball propelled by soft cilia (hairs). In a few days this ball flattens and lengthens into a fast-swimming larva covered with a ciliated velum (a sort of veil-like underwear). Soon a new bivalve shell replaces the thin larval shell and other adult organs, including a tiny foot, begin to develop. The infant mussel can creep about on solid surfaces to explore for a suitable place to anchor. This anchor consists of a strong silken thread secreted from a gland in its foot.

NAIAD. Naiads are slender-leaved aquatic plants of the family Naiadaceae that grow in freshwater ponds and lakes of temperate and tropical regions. (In Greek mythology naiads were nymphs living in and presiding over brooks, springs, and fountains.) Those that grow beneath the surface have long, gracefully waving stems, and provide shelter for many aquatic creatures.

NUDIBRANCHS (pronounced Noo'-da brangks) are found worldwide and are actually snails without a shell. They are classified as sea slugs, an unflattering term for what many consider the most beautiful animals in the sea. In deep water nudibranchs appear as colorless blobs clinging to the rocks, but in sunlit waters they flower into a fantasy of colors and seemingly limitless forms (nearly 1,000 species). Some have tentacles like rabbit ears and a rosette of gills near the rear end. Others lack gills and breathe through their skin. Some species use their gills for protection by storing in them sting cells obtained by eating other stinging animals such as sea anemones. Then, in times of danger, a number of cells are released into the water—the greater the threat, the more cells released. Nudibranchs migrate inshore to spawn and lay eggs in which the embryos develop a tiny temporary coiled shell.

OARFISH (family Regalecidae) are related to ribbonfishes. Their body structures are similar, but oarfish often reach 20 feet in length. An oarfish has a brilliant silvery body with red fins. Its two pelvic fins resemble long streamers with flattened tips like oars. The first 10 to 12 rays of its impressive dorsal fin stand plume-like on the top of its head, and the remaining shorter rays form a continuous fringe down its back to its pointed tail.

PADDLEFISH is a large, primitive sturgeon-like fish belonging to the family Polyodontidae, and the only surviving member of an order dating back 100 million years. Two freshwater species remain, one in the Mississippi basin, the other in the Yangtze river in China. It is a fierce-looking but harmless fish with a long, almost scaleless body and an extremely long paddle-like snout which it sweeps from side to side to detect plankton before opening its cavernous mouth to feed. Spawning takes place only in turbulent or flood waters and the larvae hatch from eggs, minus the paddle, which first appears in two to three weeks as a small bump.

PELICAN (*Pelecanus occidentalis*). The Brown Pelican is strictly a coastal bird and one of only two pelican species able to dive underwater for food. It fishes from Canada to southern South America and is often seen scanning the water for fish as it flies single-file in small groups close to the surface. Interestingly, each bird in the group, in order to take advantage of air currents, beats its wings sequentially in time with the bird directly in front. At times the Brown Pelican flies at greater heights; then, with half-closed wings, knifes headlong into the water with a noisy plop. It soon bobs back to the surface like a feathered cork.

PENGUIN (family Spheniscidae) is the most aquatic of all birds and lives only in cooler regions of the southern hemisphere. Penguins compensate for their inability to fly through the air by using their paddle-like wings to "fly" through the water at speeds rivaling those of seals and porpoises. All species travel swiftly by "porpoising"—that is, by alternately swimming a few yards beneath the surface, then shooting through the air like feathered missiles in a long, graceful arc before diving downward again.

PETTICOAT-FISH is one of several common names for *Gymnocorymbus ternetzi*, a strikingly colored aquarium fish originally from the Matto Grosso region of Rio Paraguay and the Rio Negro in South America. In the wild, the young live in dense shoals, swimming with military precision. The adults have olive-green backs and white undersides with a silvery sheen. A dark transverse bar extends across their eyes while the rear half of the body is gray.

PINK FAIRY, or *Mirolabrichthys tuka,* is a type of bass and a colorful reef fish of the Indo-west Pacific. Many are protogynous hermaphrodite (containing elements of both sexes, functioning first as a female, then as a male). Females are often an orange-red color, males purplish—depending on the light and the imagination of the viewer.

PIPEFISH. The family Syngnathidae comprises 150 species of unlikely looking fishes, most of which resemble 1 to 18 inch sections of garden hose. (The smallest, *Doryrhamphus melanopleura,* is much shorter than its name.) The tail fin is often fan-shaped while the head has a tubular snout that looks like a drinking straw and terminates in a tiny mouth used to suck up minute organisms. Pipefish live in tropical and temperate seas and occasionally in estuaries. Like their close relative, the sea horse, pipefish are covered with rows of bony plates instead of scales. This limits their body movement so they swim mainly with their fins. Pipefish sometimes swim horizontally and at other times vertically, heads up. Many use this vertical position to hide in clumps of eelgrass where they are hard to distinguish from their background. Following an elaborate courtship ritual, the female deposits her eggs into a brood pouch or groove on the male's underside. After incubating the eggs, the male gives birth to fully formed, thread-like offspring.

PLATYPUS is a curious looking little egg-laying mammal that appears to be made from spare parts. It has a rubbery duck-like beak, four webbed feet, and the soft fur and paddle tail of a beaver. Its streamlined 20-inch body is well adapted to life in the rivers of eastern and southern Tasmania and Australia where it lives in underwater burrows.

PUFFERFISH (family Tetraodontidae) live worldwide, mostly in the shallow waters of tropical and warm temperate seas. Most have stocky, rounded bodies, rather large eyes, and small diaphanous fins that carry them slowly through the water. While pufferfish come from a different family than balloonfish, they too can inflate themselves with water or air (even 1/4 inch long babies). However, unlike balloonfish, most puffers lack sharp spines (some have small ones) so their puffing is mostly for bluffing.

PUFFIN (*Fratercula artica)* or "sea parrot" is found in coastal areas of the northern Atlantic Ocean. Its black, white, and grey coloring, red-button eyes, red-orange feet, and a gaily colored (during the breeding season) parrot-like beak give it a whimsical appearance that belies its hardiness. Although a strong flyer in the air, it excels in flying underwater where it feeds on fish and mollusks. It spends eight months each year on the open Atlantic, then returns to its north Atlantic island birthplace to nest in burrows on the ground or on slopes. It lays a single egg and, after several weeks, abandons the tiny chick to find its way to the edge of the cliff and into the sea. Yet, according to *Life Histories of North American Birds,* parent birds have been known to hold the chick's wing tip to help it on its treacherous downward journey.

PUMPKINSEED, or *Lepomis gibbosus,* is a small freshwater sunfish shaped like its namesake and belonging to the family Centrarchidae. It is found from the Great Lakes to Texas and Florida and inhabits quiet lakes and ponds, particularly those with ample vegetation and a sandy bottom. One of two dozen perch-like species, pumpkinseed is the most colorful, especially in sunlight where it shimmers with iridescent blue and green. When building the nest, the male fans the sand with his fins to create a small hollow into which a female lays 1,000 or so eggs. He then tends to the eggs himself and, after they hatch, he guards them for about two weeks, ushering them back to the nest each night.

RAYS include several families of fish that look more like futuristic birds flying in a watery world. Their flattened bodies merge with their wings into an unbroken line to produce the characteristic diamond shape. These "wings" are actually greatly extended pectoral fins which, as in all fish, correspond to the forelimbs of the higher vertebrates. Most rays have whip-like tails tipped with poisonous spines. They inhabit both warm and temperate seas and, depending on the species, are seen near the surface or cruising silently along the sea floor.

RIBBONFISH, of the family Trachipteridae, are also aptly called sea serpents because they glide through the water in serpentine fashion. They are related to crestfish and oarfish—all having long, extremely slim, and fragile bodies. The most fragile is *Trachipterus arcticus* whose length is about 6½ feet, height 8 inches, width only 1 inch. The common name for this group in German is *Sensenfische* meaning "scythe fishes"; it refers to the first dorsal fin that looks like an upright scythe.

SAND BUG *(Hippa talpoida)* is sometimes known as the Humpty Dumpty Crab or Tadpole Crab because of its shiny and smooth, 1¼ inch long, egg-shaped carapace. *Hippa* spends its life in the wet sand at the low tide line or swimming about in tidal pools. When necessary, it can use its legs with lightning speed to shovel itself quickly into the sand and out of sight.

SAND DOLLAR belongs to the same class as the sea urchin (Echinoidea). However, its round shell is flattened and covered with short, soft spines giving it the appearance of a powder puff rather than an animal. On its upper surface is a five-petaled flower design defined by tiny perforations through which small feet protrude. Those on top are used for respiration while those on the underside aid locomotion. Its round mouth with five sharp teeth is also in the center of the underside. At low tide or to avoid a predatory starfish, sand dollars use their feet and silky spines to dig obliquely into the sand. Sand dollars are found on both coasts of the U. S. and in varying sizes. The species *Mellita testudinata* grows to about 3 inches across whereas the sand dollar-type urchin, *Clypeaster subdepressus,* lives in deep water and sometimes grows to a foot across.

SAND HOPPER (or sand flea) is a tiny, nimble-footed amphipod (a type of crustacean without a shell) that lives in the moist sand of some sea shores. Ironically, it is menaced by the water, the very element that gives it life. It is a poor swimmer and may drown if submerged too long—yet, it requires dampness and the salt to live. However, the sand hopper is endowed with a veritable tool chest of appendages for digging, jumping, culling, feeling, biting, holding, and even body brushing. It is among nature's neatest creatures, spending much time in its burrow cleaning itself. The Common Sand Hopper *(Talitrus salator)* is specially adapted for springing. By abruptly jerking its tail, it can snap along at distances several times its own length. Also, if it becomes lost, *Talitrus,* like the honey bee, has an internal compass by which it orients itself to the sun (and possibly to the moon) to find its way back.

SAWFISH (family Pristidae) live mainly on the bottom of coastal waters in all warm seas, occasionally moving into freshwater rivers and estuaries. They are named for their long, flat, saw-toothed snouts which they swing from side to side in schools of fish to stun or injure them for easier capture. However, the saw is used primarily to probe for bottom-dwelling invertebrates. Sawfish give birth to live young which are first hatched from eggs within the mother's body. Fortunately for the mother, the babies are born with soft saws.

SCALLOPS are fan-shaped bivalves (having twin shells) of the Pectinidae family. The lips of each shell half are lined with a fringe of tentacles that provides highly developed senses of touch and smell. Also spaced around the fluted edge of each shell, between the fringes, are several dozen tiny, jewel-like bright blue eyes that help it avoid the greatest enemy of all bivalves, the starfish. A scallop can swim sideward, forward, or backward (hinge first) in a lurching manner by clacking its shell halves together. It feeds by filtering minute organisms through its opened shell.

SCUD *(Gammarus locusta)* is a bug-eyed "shrimp" of a shrimp (only ½ inch long) that belongs to the order Amphipoda. Although it has no carapace and must travel about naked, it is a nimble aqua acrobat with several groups of legs, each group serving a different purpose. When not scudding along on its side or swimming on its back, this minikin can be found in wet areas between the tide lines under stones and other objects. Most amphipods carry their babies in an abdominal pouch, but a member of another suborder, the amphipod *Phronima,* is perhaps the most resourceful mother. First, she catches and eats a drifting tunicate such as a sea squirt, places her offspring in its barrel-shaped transparent shell, then pushes it along through the water like an aquatic baby carriage.

SEA CUCUMBERS are strange creatures that look more like their vegetable namesake than animals. There are 900 saltwater species living from shallow tidal areas to depths of 30,000 feet. All belong to the same diverse group as sea urchins, starfish, brittle stars, and sea lilies (phylum Echinodermata) and come in various colors. Sea cucumbers have flexible, tubular bodies with tentacle-fringed mouths at one end. Some burrow into the sand, arching their bodies so that both ends are exposed. Others lie on their sides and move about on rows of tube feet. Those without tube feet move along by alternately contracting and extending their bodies and, when necessary, by gripping the floor with their tentacles. Sea cucumbers also have remarkable defensive and regenerative powers. Some, when in danger, can eject their viscera through their posterior end, and others can twist themselves in half. In the first instance, the viscera is soon regrown, while the cucumber that was once one eventually becomes two. The Cotton Spinner sea cucumber can even bend so that its posterior faces its attacker, ready to shoot a mass of entangling threads. However, in unfavorable water currents, the "attackee" itself may become entangled.

SEA FANS belong to a group of soft corals called gorgonians because they consist of gorgonin, a tough, flexible material similar in composition to the nails and scales of vertebrates. Gorgonians in turn belong to a large group (class Anthoza) comprising over 6,000 marine species of "flower animals" of various forms and colors. Sea fans, which add flamboyant touches of color to the tropical waters they live in, grow fan-like from a central rod, branching outward in a series of interconnected flattened tubes which resemble a filagreed or lacy fan. Each tube in the fan contains hundreds of pores and each pore contains a minute polyp which is joined to the rear of its neighbor by an external tubular extension. This arrangement provides a unique communication system enabling the polyps to contract in a flash. Also, the fan can be turned broadside against the prevailing current so the mouths of the hungry polyps, fringed with stinging tentacles, can capture microscopic crustaceans.

SEA MOTH. Little is known about the biology of these curious little fish which belong to the Pegasidae family. They all have large pectoral fins that spread out in moth-like wings, and bodies covered with hard bony plates like armor. Though sea moths are now found in warmer waters in the Indo-Pacific from the east African coast to Hawaii, their existence was first discovered in Europe when they arrived as dried specimens in Chinese insect boxes. The genus *Pegasus* is blood red with blue eyes, while the armor on *Acanthopegasus'* body and head is carved in beautiful star-like designs.

SEA ROBIN is a common name for the gurnard fish from the Triglidae family that lives worldwide in tropical and temperate seas. It has large wing-like pectoral fins with two to three separate rays which it uses as fingers to probe the sand for food or when walking on the sea floor. One of many fish that make noises, the sea robin uses special muscles to contract its swim bladder to grunt, snore, cackle, or croon. It also is reputed to cackle angrily if handled roughly or, if tame, to cluck softly when stroked.

SEA SQUIRTS are so named because they squirt water when disturbed. They are members of the highly diverse phylum Chordata and are also known as tunicates. The adults are seen in a variety of colors and in numerous variations of their basic blob shape. They also have inhalant and exhalant openings through which nutrient-rich water passes. Some sea squirts live a solitary life attached to the substrate; others form colonies, while other species with transparent barrel-shaped bodies, jet freely through open waters. The offspring of sea squirts, which resemble tadpoles with rudimentary backbones, are thought to be the forerunners of higher vertebrates. They swim among the plankton and eventually settle on a hard surface to begin their metamorphosis.

One adult species, *Oikopleura*, is a unique free swimmer. It retains its larval form throughout adulthood and constructs a remarkable dwelling that doubles as an efficient feeding machine. It spins a transparent mucus bubble around itself complete with screened windows on the top, and front and back doors on the bottom. The windows admit only the tiniest morsels which are caught in filters made of fine mucus threads. To draw in nourishing currents of water, and to jet along, *Oikopleura* sits inside and undulates its tail. The water passes through the front opening and out the back, as does "Oiky" should a hasty retreat be necessary.

SEA WHIP is another exquisite marine animal in disguise that comes in many colors and forms ranging from a single long whip-like tendril to multibranched shrub-like stands. A sea whip, like the sea fan, is covered with pores, each housing a famished polyp. Each polyp, when extending its feathery tentacles, resembles a lavishly blooming flower. As with all flower-like animals, their beauty can best be observed from beneath the surface of clear waters by snorkeling, skin diving, or from a glass bottom boat. Consistent with others in their class (Anthoza), fertilization most often occurs when males and females release eggs and sperm which unite in the sea. The eggs then hatch into free swimming larvae and join the plankton community for a time before they settle to the substrate and metamorphose into adults.

SHOVELER (*Anas clypeata*) belongs to the large group of dabbling ducks and is truly a "duck for all seasons" because it is found throughout the world. It is easily recognized by its unusually long, broad, and flat bill as well as the drake's striking plumage. Shoveler loves most to dabble in freshwater bogs, marshes, streams, and ponds, churning up the mud with its bill and straining the water for snails, insects, fish, and crustaceans.

SKIMMER is one of three species of tropical birds belonging to the family Rynchopidae. It is so named because it flies low over the water, skimming the surface for fish with its long lower bill that is flattened laterally and is knife-blade thin at the tip. The American Skimmer is found only in coastlands and by the shore.

SMELTS are small silvery fish belonging to the family Osmeridae. One type, the Argentines, are saltwater fish while the Graylings, sometimes with beautiful markings, are freshwater fish found on both sides of the Atlantic.

SNAPPERS belong to a large family (Lutjanidae) of predominantly marine fish that live mostly in the warmer waters of the world. They usually live in small schools, adding bright splashes of color to the coral reefs and coastal waters. Generally, the shallow-water types tend toward yellows and greens with contrasting dots and stripes, while the deepwater versions display tones of crimson or rose. They feed mainly at night on nearly anything edible. When hunting, they first stalk their prey, then rush in to snap it up in their large, sharp-toothed mouths—hence their name. Afterwards,

they swim back to the starting point and repeat the procedure.

SPOONBILL (family Threskiornithidae). This large, long-legged wading bird, a relative of the ibis, has a long, flat spoon-like bill which it sweeps back and forth in large arcs to filter crustaceans from the water. The Roseate Spoonbill, with its flaming pink plumage, ranks among the world's most beautiful birds. It is found in Florida and South America, while the white Spoonbill lives in marshy regions, lagoons, estuaries, and seashores of Europe. Another similar version with a red face and bright pink legs lives in Africa.

SQUID, sometimes called "sea arrow" by Jacques Cousteau, includes numerous species of intelligent, fast swimming mollusks. However, the only vestiges of their molluskan heritage are a light, quill-shaped inner shell that adds stiffening to their torpedo-shaped bodies and a thick, muscular mantle that protects them as a shell protects their bottom dwelling relatives. At squid's pointed rear end is a pair of triangular fins that ripple like chiffon in a breeze to stabilize or move it slowly. At the other wider end is a large head with well-developed, image-perceiving eyes and ten suckered tentacles. For fast bursts of speed, squid shoots jets of water through its siphon, a flexible tube under its chin which it can turn instantly in the required direction. Many species can shimmer with recurring color changes as they rocket along and some (even tiny babies) can shoot clouds of inky fluid to evade predators.

STINKER is a common name for *Ircinia storbilina*, a sponge frequently seen in the shallow reefs throughout the Gulf of Mexico and the Caribbean. Its name comes from the garlicky odor emanating from its bumpy, drab, cake-shaped body which is somewhat larger than a commercial bath sponge. Stinker is one of more than 2,500 known species of sponges, all aquatic animals, most of them marine. Some sponges have amazing powers of regeneration. When their cells are passed through silk they can regroup into new sponges, each with its own species. Porous sponges serve as apartment dwellings for numerous invertebrates and some small fish. Similarly, larvae of certain shrimps enter the beautiful Venus's Flower Basket sponge, then grow too large to ever escape. The Japanese often dry these sponges and their boarders and give them as wedding gifts to symbolize togetherness.

SUNFISH. Ocean sunfish include several species of surface-living fish belonging to the family Molidae and are found in warmer seas throughout the world. *Mola mola* is said to attain a weight of 3,300 pounds. Though its scientific name *Mola* means millstone, it is also called "headfish" because its huge disc-shaped body appears to be all head. Its thick, leathery skin is colored gray, olive brown, or nearly black with a silvery sheen. *Mola mola* swims in a leisurely manner, but prefers to drift along with the current near the surface eating other slow-moving prey like jellyfish. The bodies of the tiny offspring, a mere 1/8 inch long, are studded with bony spikes. But when they are 1-inch long, they begin to assume the adults' smoother shape. The adults are said to grunt when distrubed.

SUNSTAR is a gorgeous starfish (*Solaster*) that resembles a sunburst. Its large, reddish-purple center disc is surrounded by as many as 15 lighter arms, each equipped with tube feet and a light-sensitive spot. It lives in sand from the low tide line down to 20 fathoms and is found from the arctic to the English Channel. Many species of starfish reproduce when females release their eggs into the sea, followed by sperm released by the males. The resulting offspring hatch into minute larvae that swim for a time then settle to the sea floor and metamorphose into miniature replicas of their parents.

SURFBIRD (*Aphriza virgata*) is a stocky, grayish shorebird that gets its name from the ease with which it flies over turbulent surf. It spends all but six weeks each year dining on mollusks and crustaceans along wave-washed coastlines from Alaska to Chile, then apparently disappears high in the mountains of central Alaska to breed. It reportedly migrates a distance of 24,000 miles each year.

SWEEPERS are members of a small family (Pempheridae) of reef and coastal-water fish that live mainly in the Indo-Pacific area, though some species live in tropical west-Atlantic waters. These small, deep-bodied, large-eyed fish live in schools that move in unison with precise spacing between one fish and another. They interchange leaders depending on the circumstances and respond as a group when one member is attacked.

SWORDTAIL (*Xiphophorus helleri*) is a popular aquarium fish originally found in freshwater streams, lagoons, rivers, and swamps of Mexico and Guatemala. While its colors and forms vary according to habitat, all males have a distinctive elongated lower lobe on their tail fin which gives the appearance of a sword. Remarkably, females often change into males after giving birth to several broods. The ¼ inch long offspring are born live and immediately rise to the surface to fill their swim bladders with air.

THRESHER (*Alopias vulpinis*) is a 15 to 20 foot, somewhat rare and harmless shark that is found in all oceans and is occasionally seen in coastal waters. Thresher gets its name from the manner in which it uses it unusually long tail to hunt. After herding schooling fish, such as mackerel, into a compact group, it charges into their midst, thrashing its tail to disable them before moving in to feed. Females give birth to live, fully-formed replicas of the parents.

TIP-UP (*Tringa macularia*). This is one of several local names for the Spotted Sandpiper, a shorebird that summers near lakes and streams throughout the U. S. and winters in the southern hemisphere. It is named after its curious habit of bobbing its tail up and down. It also flies closer to the surface than any other shorebird and escapes danger by diving underwater either from the surface or from the air. It can swim underwater as well as walk or run along the bottom.

TRIGGERFISH (family Balistidae) are among the sea's most beautiful beings and are found mostly in tropical coastal waters around coral reefs and grass-covered areas. From the front, their bodies appear compressed, but in profile are deep and nearly diamond shaped. Most are 1 to 2 feet long, garbed in festive, often garish colors and patterns.

TRUNKFISH (family Ostraciontidae) comprise a group of box-like fishes, many of them beautiful polychromatic works of art. Most have bright colors that apparently serve as a warning to predators that their flesh is poisonous. A trunkfish is triangular or rectangular in cross section with a flat underside and it has an inflexible suit of bony armor with openings for only the eyes, mouth, gills, and fan-shaped diaphanous fins to protrude. This armor limits its swimming ability and makes it appear to move in slow motion while its fins gyrate like little propellers. However, it gets necessary bursts of speed by vigorously fluttering its tail fin from side to side. Trunkfishes, which seldom grow to more than a foot in length, live worldwide in tropical seas and are familiar inhabitants of coral reefs and sandy bottoms. Their tiny mouths (like short segments of surgical tubing) are used to blow jets of water to churn up the sandy bottom and expose edible morsels. They also have sharp teeth for crushing coral to reach the polyps inside.

TURNSTONE (*Arenaria interpres*) is a shorebird with striking plumage and short orange legs. It is so named because it uses its bill to turn over stones and other objects to find worms, insects, and other marine invertebrates. It often feeds nonstop, tossing sand and moss about until it has dug a hole nearly the size of its plump, mottled body. It nests on the ground in Arctic regions from Alaska to Greenland and migrates as far south as Australia and New Zealand.

VENUS'S GIRDLE (*Cestum veneris*) is a ribbon-shaped marine invertebrate found in tropical and subtropical waters. It grows to at least 3 feet in length and has an almost transparent, jelly-like body fringed with iridescent blue and green cilia. Venus's Girdle swims with a rippling motion and appears as a graceful, diaphanous ribbon—a fitting adornment for the mythological Venus to wear around her waist.

WATER BEARS belong to the phylum Tardigrada, comprising at least 180 species of minute animals, most less than two-hundredths of an inch long. They have four pairs of stubby legs, each with several claws, and plump, cylindrical bodies that make them appear more like animal cracker hippopotami than bears. Found worldwide in both salt and fresh water, many live in the capillary water between sand grains. Remarkably, water bears can survive extreme changes in humidity and temperature by assuming a shriveled death-like state with no metabolism. Years later they can be revived in water, ready to feed and reproduce within hours. One is reputed to have survived storage in museums for over a hundred years, then awoke and crept out of its bed of moss.

WATER BOATMAN (also known as Boat Bug) is a common name for various aquatic insects belonging to the family Corixidae. They have long, fringed, oar-like hind legs specially adapted for swimming. When a water boatman wants to submerge, it envelops itself in a silvery bubble of air so buoyant that it must clutch onto a leaf or other object to remain submerged. It can remain submerged for long periods; then, after surfacing it breaks the bubble with its head.

WATER STRIDER is a surface-living marine insect belonging to the Gerridae family and the only species (*Halobates*) that somehow has adapted to the rigors of the waves and weather of open Atlantic and Pacific seas. With the aid of long, slender legs fringed with velvety waterproof hairs and with claws set well back from the tip, it is able to skate across the surface film of water, depressing it rather than breaking it. However, if water strider should be toppled into the sea, air bubbles adhering to hairs on its legs and underside act as an air float to help it bob right up again.

WATER WITCH is a common name for the Grebe (family Podicipedidae), a group of almost totally aquatic birds. A water witch's plumage is striking, but its short, narrow wings make it a poor flier. Conversely, it is a fast swimmer and good diver, able to evade pursuers by expelling air from its body and feathers and quickly diving underwater where it swims with its legs. It also submerges to catch tadpoles, shrimp, fish, etc. Water witches summer worldwide on reed-fringed marshes, lakes, and ponds and generally winter in saltwater areas. Their elaborate courtship ritual includes loud vocalizing, bowing, side by side running on the water's surface, and rearing and circling breast to breast while rapidly treading water. Babies ride on the backs of their parents, even during dives.

WHIRLIGIG or *Gyrinus* (family Gyrinidae) is a small, oval-shaped water beetle that resembles a slightly flattened coffee bean. It spends most of its time gyrating about like a tiny rudderless speedboat on the surface of quiet ponds, lakes, or puddles. When it dives underwater, it takes along an air bubble attached to its abdomen. The whirligig has legs specially adapted for swimming and eyes that simultaneously see above and below the surface. Its larvae offspring are cannibalistic; but, after a month of hiding and hunting on the bottom, they rise to the surface and begin to whirl around with the rest of the gang.

REFERENCES

Burton, Maurice and Burton, Robert. *Encyclopedia of Fish*. London: Octopus Books Ltd., 1975.

Carson, Rachel. *The Edge of the Sea*. New York: The New American Library, 1955.

Chromie, William J. *The Living World of the Sea*. Englewood Cliffs, NJ: Prentice-Hall, 1966.

Collins, Henry Hill, Jr. (Ed.). *Bent's Life History of North American Birds*. New York: Harper, 1960.

Grizmek, Dr. Bernhard. *Animal Life Encyclopedia*. New York: Van Nostrand Reinhold, 1974.

Hausman, Leon A. *Beginner's Guide to Seashore Life*. New York: Putnam, 1949.

Klots, Elsie B. *New Field Book of Freshwater Life*. New York: Putnam, 1966.

The New Larousse Encyclopedia of Animal Life. New York: Bonanza Books, 1981.

Nichols, David and Cooke, John A. L. *Oxford Book of Invertebrates*. Oxford University Press, 1971.

Pough, Richard H. *Audubon Water Bird Guide*. Garden City NY: Doubleday and The American Garden Guild, Inc., 1951.

Reid, George K. *Pond Life*. New York: Golden Press, 1967.

Schmitt, Waldo L. *Crustaceans*. Ann Arbor: Ann Arbor Science Library, University of Michigan Press, 1971.

Sterba, Gunther. *Freshwater Fishes of the World*. Translated and revised by Denys W. Tucker, New Jersey: T.F.H. Publications, 1973.

Tinker, Spencer Wilkie. *Fishes of Hawaii*. Honolulu: Hawaiian Service Inc., 1978.

Wheeler, Alwyne. *Fishes of the World*. New York: Macmillan, 1975.

INDEX OF AQUACISES

EMBELLISHMENTS

TERRI LEE AQUACISE® PADDLES. Strong, lightweight hand paddles specially designed for "Paddle" and "Upper Limb" Aquacises. Also useful for therapy with physician's permission. $8.00/set postpaid.

WATER WORKOUTS™ MUSICAL CASSETTE PROGRAMS. Based on Terri's student-tested Aquacises system for total-body conditioning for a firm, trim figure and healthier cardiovascular system. WATER WORKOUTS have been featured in *Vogue, Harper's Bazaar, Poolife,* and *The Journal of Physical Education and Recreation.* Simple instructions on "what" and "how" are on Side I of each cassette and in the illustrated booklet that comes with it. Side II is the fun side with 19 or more Aquacises cleverly set to special music, and cued for your nonstop exercise enjoyment. Just slip the cassette into your battery-powered (for safety's sake) player and go to it!

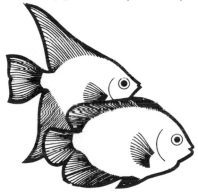

For variety, there are three different programs, each of which can be performed at low to high energy levels in waist-to-chest-deep water.

1. **DOLPHIN**—Good pace with music ranging from romantic to light and happy.

2. **FUNKY FROG**—With music ranging from slow to jaunty to fast.

3. **SUMMER RAIN**—Music ranging from romantic to bright and bouncy to lively uptempo. Program includes cardiovascular information and an easy, optional method for pulse monitoring when Aquacising aerobically.

NOTE: These programs are ideal teaching aids. Order all three, get "Tips for Teachers" free.

HINT: WATER WORKOUTS musical cassettes make novel, thoughtful gifts for friends who have a pool!

Each program (cassette and booklet) $20.00/set postpaid. Use order form on next page or write to Terri Lee, P.O. Box 5444, Scottsdale, AZ 85261.

AMERICA'S REACTION TO WATER WORKOUTS™

"I want you to know how much fun my college-age granddaughter and I have had with the cassette programs. Your *Aquacises* are for all ages!"

Arizona

"The *Aquacises* cassettes are great fun and my husband and I are now addicts to your regimen! Can't wait for *Summer Rain*. Keep them coming!"

Connecticut

"We use the cassettes for the children in our school and the seniors in our community."

Massachusetts

"We love your *Aquacises* cassettes!"

Georgia

"When I discovered your *Dolphin* tape, I got a group of my friends together to try your suggestions. We loved it! Send *Funky Frog* quickly."

Kentucky

"I love the *Water Workouts* cassettes and so do my students."

Arizona

"I've used the *Funky Frog* cassette and it works beautifully on my portable. It's a joy!"

Virginia

"I can't begin to tell you how much I have enjoyed using your tapes in our condominium pool. I usually invite several people to do the exercises and they are all as enthusiastic as I am."

Texas

"Thanks for a good daily workout!"

New York

"The ladies are loving your tapes! They use both of them (*Dolphin* and *Funky Frog*) every day."

Texas

"I have just about worn out the *Dolphin* and *Funky Frog* tapes. All of our participants WANT MORE!"

Georgia

"Stimulating, invigorating, and great fun!"

National Association of Pool Owners

232

ORDER FORM

Send to Terri Lee, P.O. Box 5444, Scottsdale, AZ 85261

Name_____
Street Number _____
City _____ State_____ Zip_____

Here's my order. I enclose $20.00 for each cassette with booklet postpaid and/or $8.00 for each set of Aquacise Paddles.

☐ DOLPHIN   ☐ FUNKY FROG   ☐ SUMMER RAIN   ☐ SET(S) AQUACISE PADDLES

Canadian customers, please remit by money order in U.S. funds.
Arizona residents, add 6.7% state sales tax.

ORDER FORM

Send to Terri Lee, P.O. Box 5444, Scottsdale, AZ 85261

Name_____   _____
Street Number _____   _____
City _____ State_____ Zip_____

Here's my order. I enclose $20.00 for each cassette with booklet postpaid and/or $8.00 for each set of Aquacise Paddles.

☐ DOLPHIN   ☐ FUNKY FROG   ☐ SUMMER RAIN   ☐ SET(S) AQUACISE PADDLES

Canadian customers, please remit by money order in U.S. funds.
Arizona residents, add 6.7% state sales tax.

ORDER FORM

Send to Terri Lee, P.O. Box 5444, Scottsdale, AZ 85261

Name_____
Street Number _____
City _____ State_____ Zip_____

Here's my order. I enclose $20.00 for each cassette with booklet postpaid and/or $8.00 for each set of Aquacise Paddles.

☐ DOLPHIN   ☐ FUNKY FROG   ☐ SUMMER RAIN   ☐ SET(S) AQUACISE PADDLES

Canadian customers, please remit by money order in U.S. funds.
Arizona residents, add 6.7% state sales tax.

BOOK REVIEWS

Publisher's Weekly

AQUACISES: Terri Lee's Water Workout Book
ISBN O-8359-O152-1

Workouts get wet with Terri Lee's **Aquacises,** and the benefits of exercising in water are convincing. Water cushions the body as it moves, thus relieving various skeletal, muscular and circulatory stresses encountered in land exercises, while acting as a resistance tool to enhance the workout. It also keeps the body from overheating, a major source of "land fatigue." Designed for nonswimmers as well as swimmers, **Aquacises** provides a complete shape-up plan, which can be pursued modestly or energetically depending on one's initial fitness level, making this appropriate for both beginning or advanced athletes, young or old. Lee's emphasis is clearly on enjoyment and getting the most out of exercise; the impressive variety of movements — illustrated by stick-figure diagrams and carefully described — assures that monotony should be no problem. Lee will also be marketing a laminated, water-proof card to be used poolside as a guide for novices, a bright idea considering the abundance of instructions this intelligent and worthwhile book contains.

Booklist

Lee, Terri. Aquacises: Terri Lee's Water Workout Book, 1984 (O-8359-O152-1)

Exercising in the water has long been therapeutic aid for the elderly, the injured, and the handicapped. The water insulates the body from many of the shocks generated by such activities as jogging or racquetball. Lee presents a huge variety of water exercises, some for specific body parts. The text is accompanied by simple but effective line drawings, many in sequence. Swimming ability is not required as many of the exercises are performed in the shallows, holding onto the pool edge, or with a flotation device. Guidelines are also included for designing a personal program. Recommended for most fitness collections.

Quincy, Patriot-Ledger, (Quincy, MA)

Aquacises: Terri Lee's Water Workout Book
by Terri Lee

In sharp contrast to the fast-buck attitude that permeates the pages of most popular fitness books, Terri Lee's **Aquacises** is utterly refreshing. Her love for the water and care for her readers and students come through loud and clear.

"Whatever the reason for the eternal fascination with our water world, it remains a respite for our gravity-heavy bodies and brings endless pleasure for all those who venture into it," she writes.

And what's more, Lee knows her stuff. Her writing shows a firm understanding of muscle science and the principles of keeping fit. Her exercises are based on 15 years of working with students in the H_2O.

Aquacises, an expanded version of a book she wrote in 1969, is a gold mine of water exercises. The book includes hundreds of exercises for strengthening and stretching the major muscles of the body. It also includes workouts with paddles, kickboards and beach balls, and tips on how to exercise aerobically in the water.

Lee emphasizes the benefits of working out in the water as opposed to on the hard, ungiving land. "Just standing chest-deep in water brings benefits," she writes.

"When in it, you are virtually free of gravity and the stress it produces on your skeletal, respiratory, digestive and circulatory mechanisms... on your entire body."

She recommends aquacises for everyone, including post-surgical patients, lap swimmers who need a break from routine and non-swimmers just getting their feet wet.

BOOK ORDER FORM

Clip and send to: Terri Lee, P.O. Box 5444, Scottsdale, AZ 85261

Please send me _____ copies of **Aquacises: Terri Lee's Water Workout Book.**

I have enclosed $22.50 for each book, postpaid, 4th class.

Arizona residents, please add 6.7% sales tax ($1.50/book). Canadian residents, please remit by money order, U.S. funds. Sorry, no C.O.D.s

Name _____
Street Number _____
City _____ State _____ Zip _____

- -

BOOK ORDER FORM

Clip and send to: Terri Lee, P.O. Box 5444, Scottsdale, AZ 85261

Please send me _____ copies of **Aquacises: Terri Lee's Water Workout Book.**

I have enclosed $22.50 for each book, postpaid, 4th class.

Arizona residents, please add 6.7% sales tax ($1.50/book). Canadian residents, please remit by money order, U.S. funds. Sorry, no C.O.D.s

Name _____
Street Number _____
City _____ State _____ Zip _____

- -

BOOK ORDER FORM

Clip and send to: Terri Lee, P.O. Box 5444, Scottsdale, AZ 85261

Please send me _____ copies of **Aquacises: Terri Lee's Water Workout Book.**

I have enclosed $22.50 for each book, postpaid, 4th class.

Arizona residents, please add 6.7% sales tax ($1.50/book). Canadian residents, please remit by money order, U.S. funds. Sorry, no C.O.D.s

Name _____
Street Number _____
City _____ State _____ Zip _____

TERRI LEE BIOGRAPHY

Terri Lee's love affair with the water began very early in life when swimming was prescribed as part of her tuberculosis rehabilitation program. Like the proverbial duck taking to water, Terri won her first Red Cross Elementary Swimmers' certificate at the age of five. She soon became an accomplished swimmer and then broadened her creative interests with eleven years of ballet instruction.

Later, as a young mother of two daughters, Terri resumed her quest for new creative outlets by studying modern dance and artistic and synchronized swimming. She also taught classes using her own unique land exercises and performed with a dance concert group. However, artistic swimming eventually became her greatest interest. Following initial artistic swimming training at a Northwestern University seminar, Terri trained under the guidance of Beulah Gundling, the world's foremost Aquatic Artist. During that time, she completed additional college courses in physical education and taught all levels of basic and synchronized swimming for YWCAs and other organizations in the east and midwest.

She also distinguished herself as an outstanding aquatic artist by winning high honors In national competitions during the 1960s. In addition, her teaching abilities and innovative methods led to invitations to conduct workshops at several aquatic symposiums and to conduct exercise programs at the Elizabeth Arden Maine Chance Farm in Augusta, Maine, and their Washington, D.C. salon.

During her years of training, teaching, and performing, Terri came to the realization that water was the ideal medium for developing total body fitness. Intrigued with its possibilities, she began to formulate a system of simple muscular and cardiovascular conditioning exercises based on the water's resistance — a concept virtually unexplored before that time.

In 1969, Terri introduced her book **Aquacises: Water Exercises for Fitness and Figure Beauty,** the first comprehensive book of aquatic exercise and the genesis of water exercise programs today. It was immediately endorsed by the President's Council on Physical Fitness and Sports and was enthusiastically received by thousands of individuals as well as colleges, universities, physical therapy and mental health organizations, retirement communities, the National YWCA, YMCA, and the Jewish Welfare Board. She also introduced her methods to the aquatic community through guest appearances at conferences for the National YWCA, CNCA (Council for National Cooperation in Aquatics); Women's National Aquatic Forum, The United States Swimming Foundation, and various universities.

In the late 1970s, she introduced three audio cassette programs, each featuring a different variety of Aquacises set to music ("Dolphin," "Funky Frog," and "Summer Rain"). However, because of her never-ending desire to explore all possibilities, she developed several new concepts for exercise in the water which she incorporated into her latest book **Aquacises: Terri Lee's Water Workout Book,** a virtual encyclopedia of aquatic movement. These efforts have created an intense interest in water exercise and a corresponding demand for a larger audio cassette library, a task Terri has met with two additional programs. "Aqua Baby" and "Aqua Sprite." More audio programs are planned for introduction in 1990-1991: "Aerobic Abalone," "Clownfish Capers," and "Ragtime Ribbonfish," as well as instructional video cassettes.

Concurrent with an active teaching schedule, Terri also serves on the Board of Directors of the United States Water Fitness Association and on its committees for Instructor Certification and Ethics for Water Fitness Instructors. Because of her ability and interest in people of all ages, she also is certified by the Metropolitan Washington Arthritis Foundation to conduct programs for "People with arthritis."

NOTES

NOTES

NOTES